AF758127

Atlas of Surgical Correction of Female Genital Malformation

Lan Zhu • Felix Wong • Jinghe Lang
Editors

Atlas of Surgical Correction of Female Genital Malformation

Springer

Editors
Lan Zhu
Obstetrics and Gynecology
Peking Union Medical College Hospital
Beijing
China

Jinghe Lang
Obstetrics and Gynecology
Peking Union Medical College Hospital
Beijing
China

Felix Wong
Obstetrics and Gynaecology
Liverpool Hospital
Liverpool
Australia

ISBN 978-94-017-7245-7 ISBN 978-94-017-7246-4 (eBook)
DOI 10.1007/978-94-017-7246-4

Library of Congress Control Number: 2015947346

Springer Dordrecht Heidelberg New York London
© Springer Science+Business Media Dordrecht 2015
This work is subject to copyright. All rights are reserved by the Publisher, whether the whole or part of the material is concerned, specifically the rights of translation, reprinting, reuse of illustrations, recitation, broadcasting, reproduction on microfilms or in any other physical way, and transmission or information storage and retrieval, electronic adaptation, computer software, or by similar or dissimilar methodology now known or hereafter developed.
The use of general descriptive names, registered names, trademarks, service marks, etc. in this publication does not imply, even in the absence of a specific statement, that such names are exempt from the relevant protective laws and regulations and therefore free for general use.
The publisher, the authors and the editors are safe to assume that the advice and information in this book are believed to be true and accurate at the date of publication. Neither the publisher nor the authors or the editors give a warranty, express or implied, with respect to the material contained herein or for any errors or omissions that may have been made.

Printed on acid-free paper

Springer Science+Business Media B.V. Dordrecht is part of Springer Science+Business Media (www.springer.com)

Contents

Contributors

Li Bin Department of Obstetrics and Gynecology, An Zhen Hospital, Subsidiary of Capital Medical University, Beijing, China

Juan Chen Department of Obstetrics and Gynecology, Peking Union Medical College Hospital, Beijing, P. R. China

Na Chen Department of Obstetrics and Gynecology, Peking Union Medical College Hospital, Beijing, P. R. China

Qing Dai Department of Ultrasound, Peking Union Medical College Hospital, Beijing, P. R. China

Limin Feng Department of Gynaecology, Beijing Tiantan Hospital, The Capital University of Medical Sciences, Beijing, China

Xianghua Huang Department of Obstetrics and Gynecology, The Second Hospital of Hebei Medical University, Shijiazhuang, Hebei, China

Fang Jiang Department of Obstetrics and Gynecology, Peking Union Medical College Hospital, Beijing, P. R. China

Hang Mei Jin Department of Obstetrics, Affiliated Obstetrics and Gynecology Hospital, College of Medical Sciences, Zhejiang University, Hangzhou, China

Jingjing Lu Department of Radiology, Peking Union Medical College Hospital, Beijing, P. R. China

Xiaochuan Li Department of Obstetrics and Gynecology, Peking Union Medical College Hospital, Beijing, P. R. China

Guangnan Luo Department of Obstetrics and Gynecology, The Luohu Hospital of Shenzhen, Shenzhen, China

Qinjie Tian Department of Obstetrics and Gynecology, Peking Union Medical College Hospital, Beijing, P. R. China

Jiali Tong Department of Obstetrics and Gynecology, Peking Union Medical College Hospital, Beijing, P. R. China

Shu Wang Department of Obstetrics and Gynecology, Peking Union Medical College Hospital, Beijing, P. R. China

Sumin Wang Department of Obstetrics and Gynecology, Nanjing Maternity and Infant Hospital of Nanjing Medical University, Nanjing, Jiangsu, P. R. China

Huan-ying Wang Department of Obstetrics and Gynecology, An Zhen Hospital, Subsidiary of Capital Medical University, Beijing, China

Qiushi Wang Department of Obstetrics and Gynecology, The Second Hospital of Hebei Medical University, Shijiazhuang, Hebei, China

Xue Xiang Department of Gynaecology and Obstetrics, The Second Affiliated Hospital, Medical School of Xi'an Jiaotong University, Xi'an, China

Feng Xu Department of Obstetrics and Gynecology, Nanjing Maternity and Infant Hospital of Nanjing Medical University, Nanjing, Jiangsu, P. R. China

Jie Yang Department of Obstetrics and Gynecology, Peking Union Medical College Hospital, Beijing, P. R. China

Huimei Zhou Department of Obstetrics and Gynecology, Peking Union Medical College Hospital, Beijing, P. R. China

Lan Zhu Department of Obstetrics and Gynecology, Peking Union Medical College Hospital, Beijing, P. R. China

Chapter 1
Abnormal Development of the Female Genital Tract

Juan Chen, Fang Jiang, Jiali Tong, and Lan Zhu

1.1 The Development of the Female Genital System

Jiali Tong, Juan Chen, and Lan Zhu

1.1.1 Anatomy of the Female Reproductive System

The female reproductive system is composed of the internal and external genitalia depending on their anatomical positions along the genital tract. The internal genitalia consist of ovaries, fallopian tubes, uterus, and vagina; the external genitalia include the mons pubis, labia majora and minora, clitoris, vestibule, and perineum. The development of these organs prior to puberty is very slow; after puberty, the follicle-stimulating hormone (FSH), luteinizing hormone (LH), and other sex hormones actively promote a rapid development of both internal and external genitalia. The uterus starts to enlarge at the age of 10, and it reaches adult size at the age of 18. The endometrium undergoes cyclical changes and sheds as menstruation under the influence of ovarian hormones. The vagina becomes long and wide and changes to gray in color. The vulva becomes swollen with pubic hairs appearing and undergoes transition to the adult appearance. The labia become hypertrophied and pigmented.

J. Chen • F. Jiang • J. Tong • L. Zhu (✉)
Department of Obstetrics and Gynecology, Peking Union Medical College Hospital,
No. 1 Shuaifuyuan, Beijing 100730, P. R. China
e-mail: zhu_julie@sina.com

© Springer Science+Business Media Dordrecht 2015
L. Zhu et al. (eds.), *Atlas of Surgical Correction of Female Genital Malformation*,
DOI 10.1007/978-94-017-7246-4_1

1.1.1.1 Internal Genitalia

Ovaries

Ovaries are the most important female sex glands. They are white, flat oval bodies of 4×3×1 cm in size, situated on both sides of the uterus. They produce ova and female hormones. They are small and smooth before 8 years old, but they begin to develop at the age of 8–10; thereafter they increase in a linear fashion. At menarche, the weight of an ovary is only 30 % of its adult's weight. It continues to increase in size and is mature at the age of 17–18. There are two aspects of ovarian development: (a) it produces germ cells and then ova, and (b) it produces sex hormones including estrogen and progesterone. Therefore, ovaries are both female reproductive organs and endocrine organs.

Fallopian Tubes

They are a pair of elongated hollow tubes lined with smooth muscles. The medial end communicates with the corner uteri and its lateral end is free lying next to the ovary. The outer end is funnel shaped with many fingerlike projections called tubal fimbria, stretching over the ovary. The fimbria helps to pick up the ovum into the fallopian tube where fertilization takes place when the sperm meets the ovum. The fertilized ovum then travels down into the uterine cavity, and then egg implantation takes place in the uterus.

Uterus

The uterus situates at the center of the pelvic cavity like an inverted pear. It measures about 7–8 cm long, 4–5 cm wide, and 2–3 cm thick. The uterus lay in an anteverted position suspended by its ligaments. Its lower one-third is the narrow cervix, which connects to the vagina. Its upper two-thirds is wider and is the uterine body. The top of the uterine body is the fundus with uterine corners on both sides and connects with a fallopian tube on each side. The cervical canal is a narrow tube-like, leading to the uterine cavity. The uterus is the breeding ground of the fetus, where pregnancy takes place. The uterus composes of three layers of tissues: (1) The inner endometrial layer is rich in glands and blood supply; the endometrium continues to change following each menstrual cycle and the woman's age. During menstruation, the shedding of the endometrium is a major component of the menses; (2) the middle layer is a very thick muscle layer. It can produce strong contractions during labor and at orgasms. It is resilient and can stretch sufficiently to accommodate a mature fetus; (3) the outermost layer is a serosal layer which is a part of the peritoneum.

Vagina

It is a soft elastic hollow tube which tilts backward. It is the female organ of sexual intercourse. It also serves as the passage of menstrual blood and the birth channel. It has a strong stretching property. With advancing age, the vaginal wall gets thinner with reducing vaginal wrinkles and weakened elasticity. Vaginal nerve endings mainly distribute in the outer 1/3 of the vagina, with no nerve endings at the upper 2/3. Therefore, the sex-sensitive area is located at the outer ½ of the vagina.

1.1.1.2 External Genitalia

Female external genitalia consist of the mons pubis, labia, and vaginal opening. All together, they are labeled as the vulva.

Mons Pubis

It is the swelling in front of the pubic symphysis, with the labia majora on adjacent sides. There are pubic hairs on the mons pubis, mostly trapezoid, inverted triangle, or rectangle in distribution. It regulates the local temperature and buffers the body impact of collision. The subcutaneous fat tissue underneath the mons pubis possesses shock-cushioning effect.

Clitoris

The clitoris is homologous to the male penis, both evolved from the same embryonic tissue. It is the only organ without reproductive function in the female genitalia, but it is related to sexual arousal and sexual function in humans. The clitoris is rich in nerve endings, which are very sensitive to touch, and it is the most important sex-sensitive zone.

Labia

There are two pairs of female labia – the labia majora and labia minora. The labia majora are the fat pads on both sides of the vaginal opening, with its skin covering with pubic hairs. Both the labia majora and minora have thin mucosal layers with no pubic hairs on its inner side. The sizes of labia and their thickness vary widely which are not directly related to sexual function. However, the labia are rich in nerve fibers and can have an important role in sexual stimulation and sexual arousal.

Vaginal Vestibule

It is a diamond-shaped area between the two labia minora. Its anterior end has the urethra where urine can pass out; its posterior has the vaginal opening with vestibular bulbs on its sides.

Bartholin Gland

Bartholin glands are located in the lower part of the labia minora as a small pair of glands, with its glandular opening between the labia minora and the hymen. If infected with inflammation, they can be significantly enlarged.

Hymen

Covering the vaginal opening is a layer of thin membrane, called "hymen." The hymen has a central hole, which varies in sizes depending on individuals. Some are too small in size, which will not allow even a finger to pass through, but others may accommodate two fingers through it. The hymen thickness is generally about 2 mm. But individuals may have very thin hymen, which may rupture during strenuous exercise or inadvertent collision to the vulva. It usually tears open at the time of first sexual intercourse and is accompanied by a small amount of bleeding.

1.1.2 The Development of the Female Reproductive System

The genetic sex of an embryo is determined by the sperm type (23X or 23Y) which fertilizes the ovum, but before 6 weeks of life, both male and female embryos have the same undifferentiated gonads, known as the undifferentiated genital phase. At the 7th week, gonads begin to have gender-related morphological changes. In the 8th to 9th weeks, internal genital differentiation begins. The external genital differentiation can only be identified at the 12th week. Therefore, the reproductive system including the gonads, reproductive tract, and external genitalia has an undifferentiated and differentiated phases of development.

1.1.2.1 The Undifferentiated Sex Phase

The Formation of the Undifferentiated Gonads

When the embryo is at 3–4 weeks' gestation, there are many reproductive cells which are larger and more round than the somatic cells lying at the posterior wall of the yolk sac near the allantoic endoderm. These are the primordial germ cells. When the embryo is at the 4th week, the sides of the embryo body start to have fold formation;

the ventral mesoderm gradually moves toward the body separated from intermediate body, forming into the left and right cord-like structure, known as nephrogenic cords. At the end of the 4th week, the volume of the nephrogenic cords continues to increase, and from the posterior wall of the embryo, it bulges to form a body cavity. At this time, at the back of the body cavity, the epithelial hyperplasia of each side of the body forms two longitudinal ridges, known as the urogenital ridges, which are the origins of kidneys, gonads, and primitive reproductive tract. In its further development, a central longitudinal groove forms in this urogenital ridge, dividing it into inner and outer parts. The outer part is longer and thicker and known as the mesonephric ridge; the inner part is shorter and thinner known as the genital ridge. When the embryo is at the 5th week, the genital ridge is covered with a layer of columnar epithelium, also called the germinal epithelium. When the embryo is at the 6th week, the germinal epithelium will hollow down and grow rapidly forming multiple cords with vertical extensions stretching between the gonadal tissues. It is also known as primary sex cord. In a 6-week embryo, primordial germ cells along the hindgut mesentery move to the genital stroma at the 10th thoracic vertebral level. The migration takes 1 week to complete. Some of these sex cord cells will surround each primordial germ cell. The larger primordial germ cells, the smaller primitive sex cord cells and the surrounding stromal tissues will form the undifferentiated gonadal tissue. At this time, whether it is a testis or an ovary cannot be distinguished. Thus, the gonads mainly come from the genital ridge of the coelomic cavity epithelium. But the epithelium, the underneath mesenchymal tissue, and the primordial germ cells are from three different origins.

The Formation of the Primitive Reproductive Tract

The development of the primitive reproductive tract is slightly later than the undifferentiated gonads. At a 6-week embryo, both male and female embryos consist of mesonephric ducts and paramesonephric ducts which are two different reproductive tracts. Both develop from the mesonephric ridge lateral to the genital ridge. One is called the mesonephric duct (also known as Wolffian duct), which originates from the mesonephros of the pronephros and gradually moves downward and ends into the primitive cloaca. This is the primitive male reproductive tract. The other is the paramesonephric duct, also called the Müllerian duct. This is the female primitive reproductive tract which forms at the time of mesonephric duct formation, at the inner aspect of mesonephric duct. It is formed by invagination of the coelomic epithelium. The upper part of the duct is located at the outer aspect of the mesonephric duct, lying parallel to each other. The middle part of the duct turns to the inner aspect and crosses the back of the mesonephric duct and lies in the inner aspect of it. In the lower end, the right and left paramesonephric ducts merge at the midline. The upper part of the paramesonephric duct has a funnel-shaped opening to the coelomic cavity forming the fimbrial end of the fallopian tube. The lower ends are blind ends merging into the sides of the back wall of the urogenital sinus. At the sinus, it forms a protrusion, called sinus tubercle, also known as the Müllerian tubercle or Müllerian nodules.

Embryonic Formation of the External Genitalia

When the embryo is at 9 weeks old, its external genitalia does not show any sex differentiation. At about the 5th week, both sides of the primordial urogenital sinus organize into folds and merge at the cephalic end forming a genital tubercle. A urorectal septum separates the cloacal opening from the primordial urogenital sinus in front and the anus at the back. Lateral to the urogenital fold, a pair of large uplift develops, forming the labia or scrotum. Urogenital fold forms a depression for a urethral groove covered by a urogenital membrane. At the 7th week, the urogenital membrane ruptures.

1.1.2.2 The Differentiated Sex Phase

Differentiation and Descending of the Gonad

The undifferentiated gonad has the potential to differentiate into the testes or ovaries. The sex differentiation depends on whether there is any testis-determining factor – TDF in the Y chromosome. At current knowledge, the Y chromosome sex-determining region Y gene – SRY – is the best candidate gene for TDF. It is situated at the short arm of the Y chromosome near the centromere in the IAIA District (Yp11.32). It contains an exon, is of a non-intron structure, and harbors the histocompatibility Y antigen – H-Y antigen.

If the membranes of body cells and primordial germ cells do not contain the H-Y antigen, the undifferentiated gonad will develop into an ovary. When the embryo is 10 weeks old, the embryonic sex cord will grow deeper, forming an incomplete ovarian network. Later, these embryonic sex cord and ovarian network will degenerate and be replaced by blood vessels and stroma forming the ovarian medulla. Thereafter, the genital surface epithelium (also known as primitive cortical cells) continues to grow thicker. It also penetrates into the deep layer, forming new cell cords, known as secondary sex cord or cortical cord. They are shorter and scatter in the cortex. In a 16th-week human embryo, cortical cord will break into many isolated cell groups that are primitive follicles, also known as primordial follicles. At this time, the ovaries are formed. Each primordial follicle has a primitive germ cell which will differentiate into a cell called oogonium.

The oogonium is surrounded by a layer of cortical cells which differentiate into small and flat follicular cells, also known as granular cells. Between the follicles mesenchymal cells differentiate into ovarian stroma. In the embryonic stage, the oogonium can split, divide, and proliferate into oocytes. There are up to six million oogonia in both ovaries. After the embryo is at the 20th week, these oogonia will no longer divide and a large number of them undergo degradation. Only some grow up and differentiate into primary oocytes. At birth, all oogonia within the ovaries disappeared, leaving about 70–200 million primary oocytes. All cells enter the first meiosis and stop dividing at their early stage. Not until after puberty, they complete their meiotic division before ovulation. Primary oocyte cannot self-replicate. After birth the primary oocytes within the ovary no longer grow, instead many of them gradually degenerate and undergo atresia. At adolescence, there are about four million remaining oocytes. After the embryo reaches 16 weeks, the ovarian cortex and medulla continue to develop. The cortical surface has a layer of connective tissue called the tunica albuginea. Outside the albuginea, it is covered by a layer of cuboidal epithelium arising from the body cavity called the ectodermal epithelia.

The ovary is initially located in the upper part of the posterior coelomic wall between the end of gonadal cord to the labia majora along a cord-like structure called ovarian gubernaculum. With the proliferation and differentiation of the gonadal cord, the gubernaculum gradually rises to the coelomic cavity and position the ovaries in the abdominal cavity. As the embryo gradually grows up, the ligament continues to shorten. The ovaries come down to a pelvic location slightly below the pelvic rim at the 12th week of gestation.

The Evolution of the Internal Genitalia

If the undifferentiated gonads differentiate into ovaries, in the absence of testes to produce androgens and no influence from any Müllerian inhibiting factor (MIF), the mesonephric ducts (Wolffian) will degenerate. The paramesonephric ducts differentiate and develop into the internal female genitalia. It is noteworthy that about 1/4 of the women may have the residual remnant of the mesonephric ducts or tubules. For example, they form the epoophoron and paroophoron in the mesovarium and the Gartner's duct cyst alongside the uterus and vagina.

But in the process of paramesonephric duct differentiation into the internal female genitalia, the mesonephric ducts and ovaries played a leading induction role. The mesonephric ducts induce the fusion and resorption of the bilateral Müllerian ducts. The ovarian tissue attached to the Müllerian duct is composed of muscle fibers from non-Müllerian and mesonephric duct origin and promotes the integration and development of the uterus.

Uterus and Fallopian Tubes

When the fetus is at about the 9th week of gestation, the upper part of the paramesonephric ducts becomes the fallopian tubes. The middle part to the lower part merges at the midline to form the uterus, the cervix, and the vaginal dome. At the beginning of the merger, there is a septum to divide into two ductal cavities. Toward the end of 12 weeks, the septum disappeared into a single cavity to form the uterus and the vaginal tube. The endometrial cavity is lined with columnar epithelium, and in the part of the uterus formed by the paramesonephric duct, the mesenchymal tissue surrounding it will proliferate actively, and the uterine wall will become thickened. The tissue at the uterine cervix will form the vaginal dome. At the 16th week, the muscular and serosal layers of the uterus will form. At the 24th week, glandular buds will form in the endometrial cavity. In the last 12 weeks, by the influence of the placental hormones, there is a rapid development of the uterus, and the endometrium will thicken and be congested with blood. At birth, the development of endometrial glands has been more mature and complete. At birth, the uterus surface is flat. The ratio of the uterine body and uterine cervix is about 1:2, until after puberty, the ratio starts to change. The uterus will further develop and mature.

The Vagina

The vagina comes from two origins. The upper 3/4 to 4/5 of the vagina is from the paramesonephric duct and the lower 1/5 to 1/4 from the urogenital sinus. At the 9th week of gestation, the caudal end of the paramesonephric duct and the back of urogenital sinus will form the paramesonephric duct tubercle (Müllerian tubercle), which is also known as the sinus tubercle. The urogenital sinus epithelial cells and cells at the caudal ends of the paramesonephric duct proliferate together and form a solid sinovaginal bulk and further develop into a vaginal plate. The vaginal plate is initially a solid tubular structure called sinovaginal bulk. It gradually expands and increases the distance between the uterus and the urogenital sinus.

From the 11th week onward, the cells in the central part of the vaginal plate gradually degenerate, forming a cavity. At the 20th week, a vagina is formed, which links the uterus internally and externally with the urogenital sinus, separated by a hymen.

In recent years, many embryologists believe that the whole vagina is from the sinovaginal bulk. The belief is that when the paramesonephric duct reaches the urogenital sinus surface and becomes surrounded by the sinovaginal bulk, the sinovaginal bulk will grow cranially and develop into the vaginal plate, as the prototype of the future vagina. After that, the vaginal plate cavitates from a top-down direction to make the vagina a top-down funnel-shaped cavity. The top forms a vaginal dome, and the bottom separates from the urogenital sinus by a thin tissue. The central part of this thin tissue will be absorbed, and it forms a hole in the vaginal hymen. Although the paramesonephric ducts do not involve in the formation of the vagina, it plays an inducing role in the evolutionary development of the sinovaginal bulk. One side of the paramesonephric duct will induce the vagina formation from the ipsilateral side. However, this belief requires future validation. Another theory is that the mesonephric duct degenerates from top downward; its end at the level of the external cervical opening enlarges to form the sinovaginal bulk and integrates with Müllerian tubercle of the paramesonephric duct. Their further proliferation will form the vaginal plate.

The Development of the External Genitalia

At the 7th to 8th week of fetal development, the external genitalia start to differentiate into male or female. When the gonad is an ovary, the body produces no testosterone. The genital tubercle gradually enlarges slowly and forms the clitoris. The urogenital folds on both sides will not merge and form the labia minora. The right and left labia fuse with the scrotal bulge in the front of the clitoris, forming the mons pubis. The posterior labia fuse together and form the posterior commissure. The rest of the non-fused labia become the labia majora. At this time, the urethral groove expands with the lower end of the urogenital sinus to form the front of the vagina. When the fetus is at the 12th week, the female external genitalia begin to take shape, and they gradually further developed.

1.2 Abnormal Development of Female Reproductive Organs

Fang Jiang, and Lan Zhu

The development and differentiation processes of the female reproductive organs are influenced by both endogenous factors (nondisjunction of the germ cell chromosomes, chimera, karyotype abnormalities, etc.) and exogenous factors (use of hormone, drugs, etc.). The differentiation of the primitive gonad, its development and fusions within the reproductive system, and cavity development and formation of the external genitalia may be affected by these factors resulting in a variety of developmental anomalies.

Abnormal development of the female reproductive organs includes the developmental and morphological anomalies in the fallopian tubes, uterus, vagina, and vulva. These anomalies can be associated with abnormal ovaries, kidney, or other organs. Most of the female genital tract anomalies arise from the developmental anomalies of the paramesonephric ducts (Müllerian duct); however, these Müllerian anomalies originate from the abnormal development of the Gartner's duct. Genital tract anomalies have different clinical manifestations. Some do not present with any clinical symptoms, others have different symptoms at different times and different ages, and the impact on fertility is also widely variable. The management of these genital anomalies varies widely from observation to surgery. Therefore, a correct diagnosis within a clear classification of these congenital anomalies is very important.

1.2.1 *The Classification of Female Reproductive Tract Anomalies*

There are many classifications of female reproductive tract anomalies. The early classification began in 1842; it is based on the embryology and Müllerian duct development, since then there are many other classifications. Before 1950, all classifications are based on embryonic developments: the Müllerian duct fusion and its abnormal developments. After 1950, the classifications take into account many other factors. This chapter describes three types of classifications for reproductive tract anomalies.

1.2.1.1 American Fertility Society (AFS) Classification of Reproductive Tract Anomalies

American Fertility Society (AFS) developed this classification in 1988 [1]. The classification is as follows [6]: (1) Anomaly caused by developmental anomaly of the Müllerian duct including the agenesis of the uterus and vagina and is a defect characterized by no reproductive potential, e.g., in the case of congenital absence of the vagina [7]. (2) Anomaly caused by the developmental anomaly of the genitourinary sinus: The urogenital sinus was not involved in the formation of the lower vagina; it is mainly responsible for the different degrees of vaginal atresia [8]. (3) Anomaly caused by abnormal fusion of the Müllerian ducts. The anomalies are divided into vertical fusion and lateral fusion anomalies. Vertical fusion anomaly presents as transverse vaginal septum and lateral fusion anomaly as longitudinal vaginal septum and oblique vaginal septum syndrome.

AFS classification is mainly based on Müllerian anomalies and their effects on fertility; it includes seven categories (Fig. 1.1): (1) Müllerian agenesis (absent uterus) or hypoplasias, (2) unicornuate uterus (a one-sided uterus), (3) uterus didelphys (double uterus), (4) bicornuate uterus (uterus with two horns), (5) septated uterus (uterine septum or partition), (6) arcuate uterus, and(7) DES uterus as a result of fetal exposure to diethylstilbestrol. This classification is simple and clear; therefore, it has been widely adopted in the past 20 years. This classification defines different levels of uterine anomalies, and its prognosis has a good clinical correlation with the pregnancy outcome. However, this classification has its limitations: Many complex reproductive tract anomalies are not covered. Category 1 includes all patients with dysplasia or congenital absence of the vagina, cervix, uterus, and/or gonads as a single class which would be too vague and generalized.

Figure 1.1 [2]

A type: bilateral developmental anomalies. (1) Vaginal agenesis, complete; (2) vaginal agenesis, partial (upper or lower); (3) cervical aplasia; (4) cervical hypoplasia; (5) tubal aplasia; (6) uterine aplasia; (7) uterine hypoplasia (with or without uterine cavity); (8) combined dysplasia

B type: unilateral developmental anomalies. (1) Unicornuate, no horn; (2) unicornuate, non-fused, non-cavitary horn; (3) unicornuate, fused, non-cavitary horn; (4) unicornuate, cavitary, non-fused horn; (5) unicornuate, cavitary, fused, noncommunicating horn; (6) unicornuate, cavitary, fused, communicating horn.

C type: fusion anomalies. (1) Vaginal septum; (2) arcuate uterus; (3) septate uterus, partial; (4) septate uterus, complete to external os of the cervix; (5) septate uterus, complete, up to internal os of the cervix; (6) complete septate, vagina, and uterus; (7) bicornuate uterus, complete to internal os of cervix; (8) bicornuate uterus, partial; (9) uterus didelphys bicollis; (10) uterus didelphys with the vaginal septum; (11) uterus didelphys with the vaginal septum, with unilateral vaginal obstruction; (12) uterus didelphys with the vaginal septum with bilateral obstructed vagina

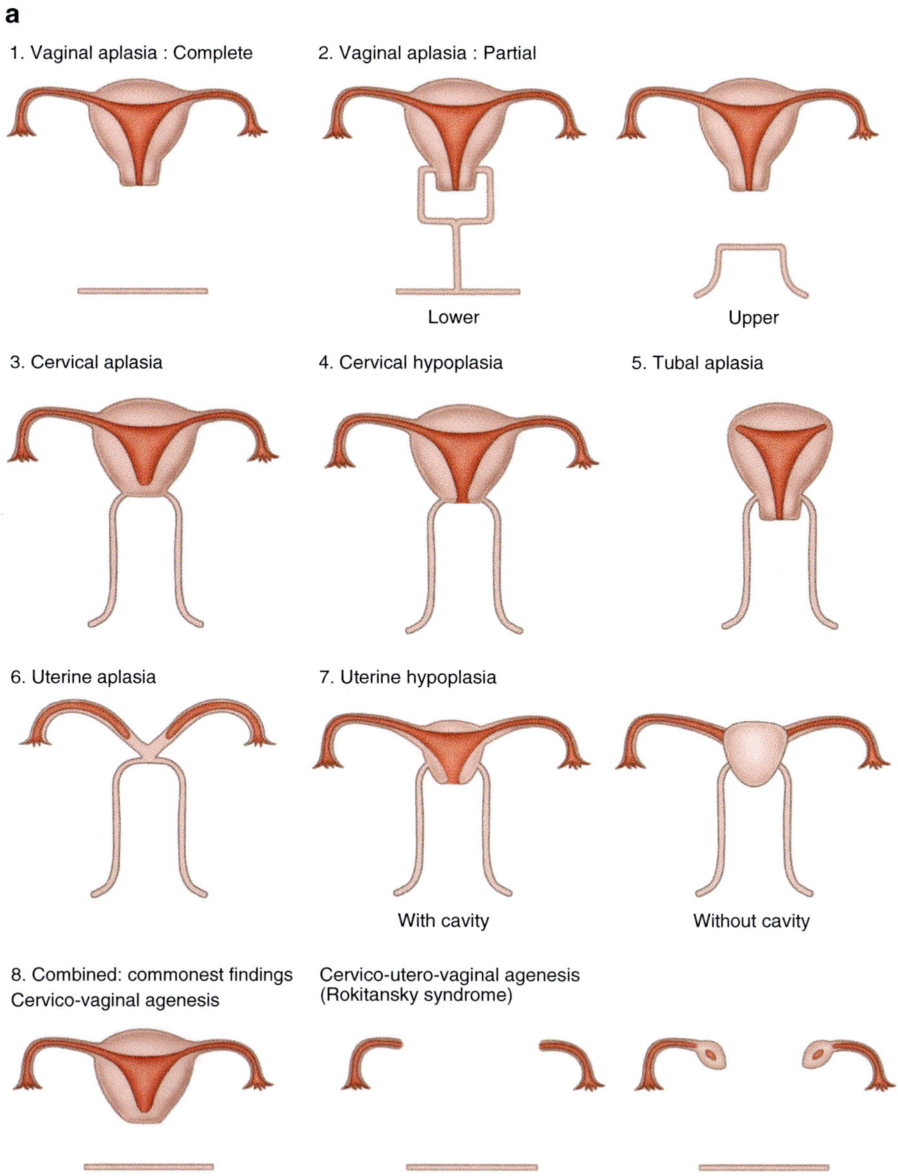

Fig. 1.1 AFS classification based on Müllerian anomalies

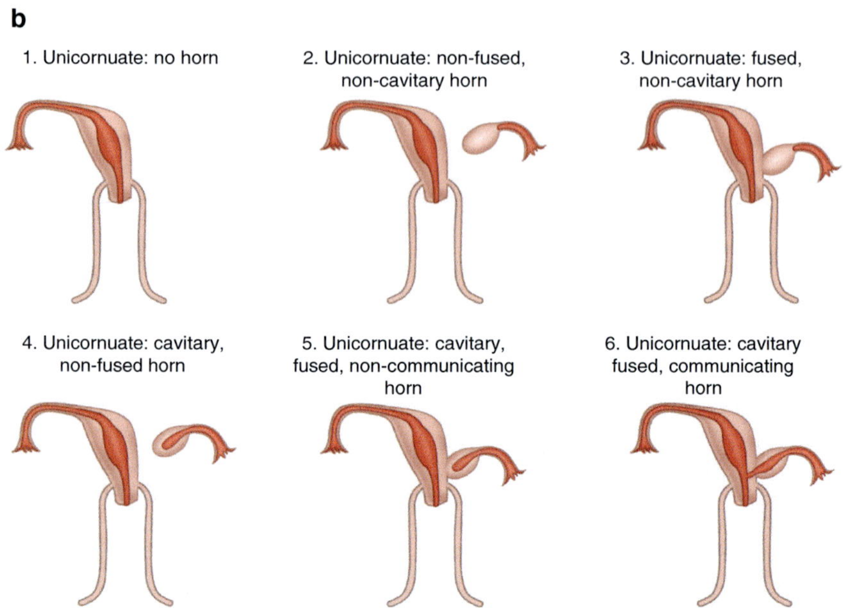

Fig. 1.1 (continued)

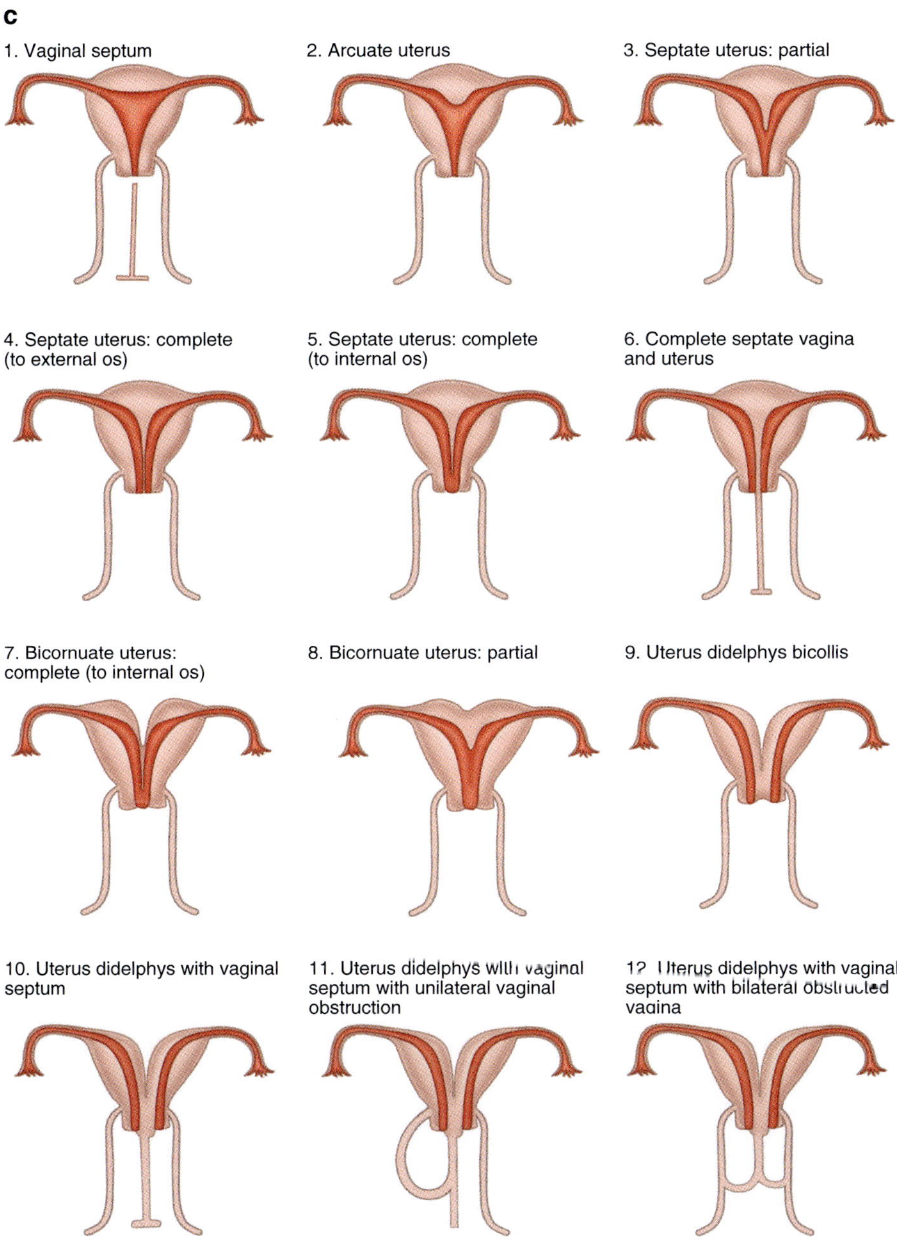

Fig. 1.1 (continued)

1.2.1.2 Acién Classification of Reproductive Tract Anomalies

In 2011, Acién [3] conducted a systematic review of relevant articles of reproductive tract anomalies from 64 full-text articles and more than 300 related clinical papers in the literature. Based on the experience gained from the application of the current classification systems and the appropriate treatment, he updated the female urogenital tract anomalies in accordance with the etiopathogenesis and proposed a new embryological-clinical classification of female reproductive tract anomalies. The system also considers both Müllerian and renal tubular developmental anomalies (Fig. 1.2), but his classification system has only been published for a short time and has not been widely used.

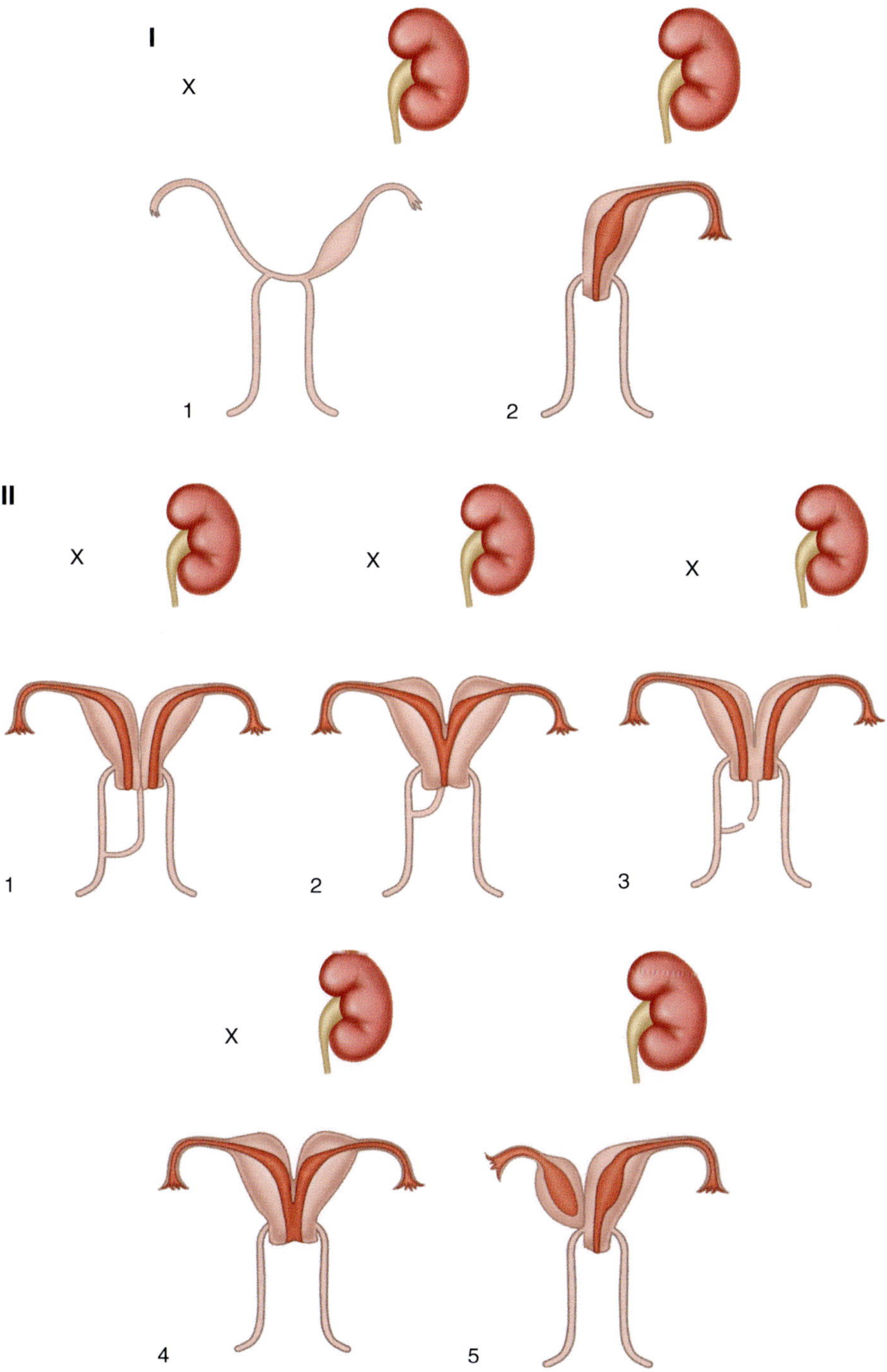

Fig. 1.2 Acién classification of reproductive tract anomalies

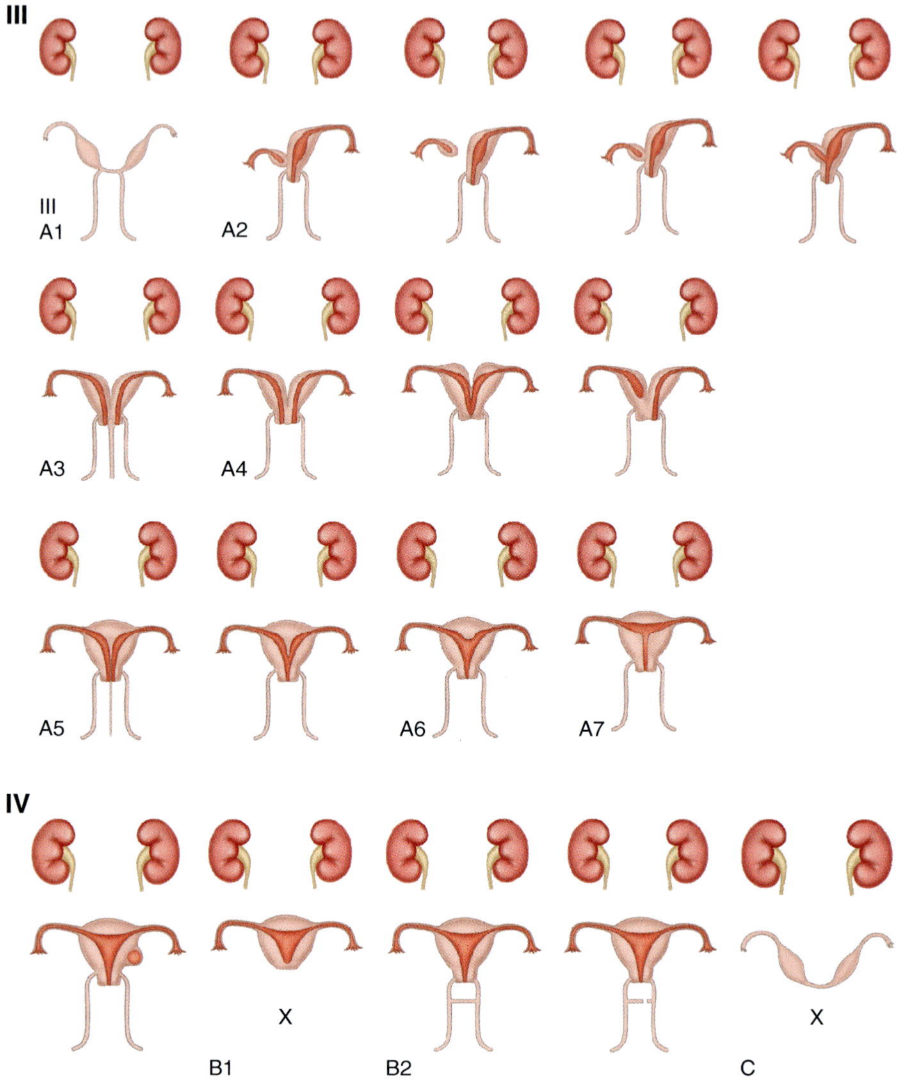

Fig. 1.2 (continued)

1.2.1.3 The European Society of Human Reproduction and Embryology (ESHRE) and the European Association for Gynaecological Endoscopy (ESGE) Classification of Female Reproductive Tract Anomalies

In 2013 the European Society of Human Reproduction and Embryology (ESHRE) and the European Association for Gynaecological Endoscopy (ESGE) proposed a new classification system based on anatomy. Anomalies are classified into the following main classes from the same embryological origin: the uterus, cervix, and vagina [4]: (Fig. 1.3).

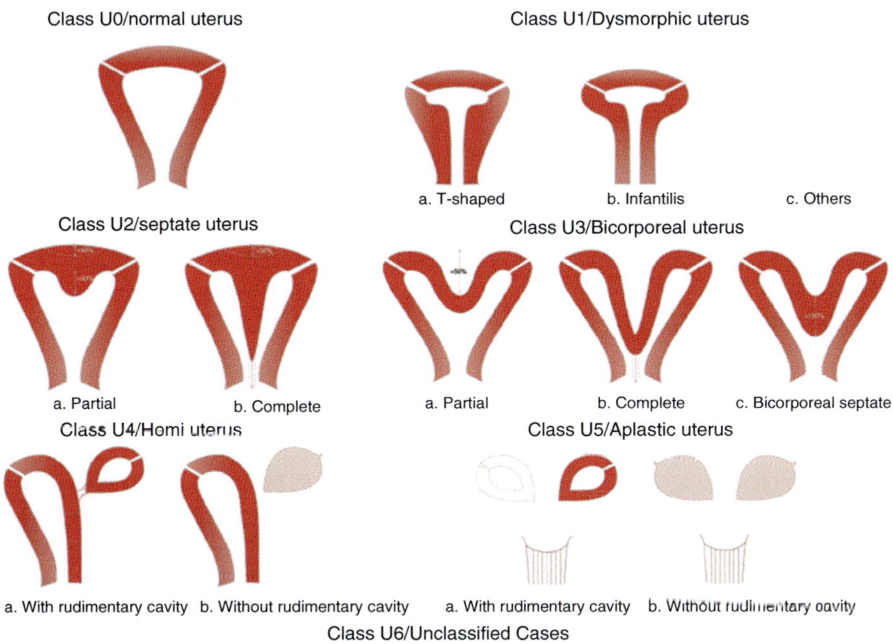

Fig. 1.3 ESHRE/ESGE – uterine anomalies

1.2.2 Common Reproductive Tract Anomalies

The current classifications of reproductive tract anomalies vary with advantages and disadvantages for each classification. Among them, there are many various nomenclatures, leading to a lot of confusion and overlapping. Hereby we describe some common reproductive tract anomalies and their clinical manifestations as follows.

1.2.2.1 External Genital Anomalies

The most common female external genital anomaly is the congenital hymen anomaly.

Congenital Hymen Anomaly

The hymen is a layer of mucosal membrane located at the vaginal opening, with squamous epithelium covering on its outer and inner surfaces. In between these surfaces it contains connective tissue, blood vessels, and nerve endings. During its development, abnormal cavity formation at the urogenital sinus will develop into various anomalies which include the imperforate hymen, microperforate hymen, septate hymen, cribriform hymen, etc. (Fig. 1.4).

Imperforate hymen is a rare genital anomaly, also known as nonporous hymen. The incidence of imperforate hymen is about 0.015 %. Imperforate hymen mainly obstructs the discharge of vaginal secretions. It may be asymptomatic at childhood due to minimal vaginal secretions, but at puberty, as both the vaginal and cervical secretions gradually increase, they accumulate in the vagina and lead to a sense of heaviness in the lower abdomen. After menarche, as the menstrual blood cannot drain out, it accumulates in the vagina forming a vaginal hematoma after several menstruations. Subsequently, it may lead to uterine and tubal hematomas, and eventually retrograde menstrual flow will enter into the pelvic cavity forming pelvic hematomas. Clinical symptoms are cyclical lower abdominal pains which progressively increase in intensity. On gynecological examination a bulging hymen can be seen, with a purple blue surface; on rectal examination, a vaginal mass bulging into the rectum is felt as a palpable pelvic mass. With a finger in the rectum, the pressing on the vaginal mass will make the bulging hymen more obvious. Ultrasound scan may show accumulated fluid in the vagina and even in the uterine cavity.

The clinical manifestations in patients with imperforate hymen or micropore hymen would vary according to the absence or sizes of the pore holes in the hymen. Some patients have periodic menstruations with moderate amount of menstrual blood outflow, but a lot of blood still accumulates in the vagina; sometimes these periods are irregular; some patients present with delayed menarche, with complaints of periodic abdominal pain, dyspareunia, and smelly vaginal discharge due to poor vaginal drainage. Similar to imperforate hymen, micropore hymen can cause the reflux of vaginal secretions and blood into the peritoneal cavity forming a pelvic mass. The micropore openings in the hymen may serve as communicating channels between the vagina and the outside, through which bacteria will enter and exit, leading to recurrent urinary tract infection and more commonly pelvic infection or abscess.

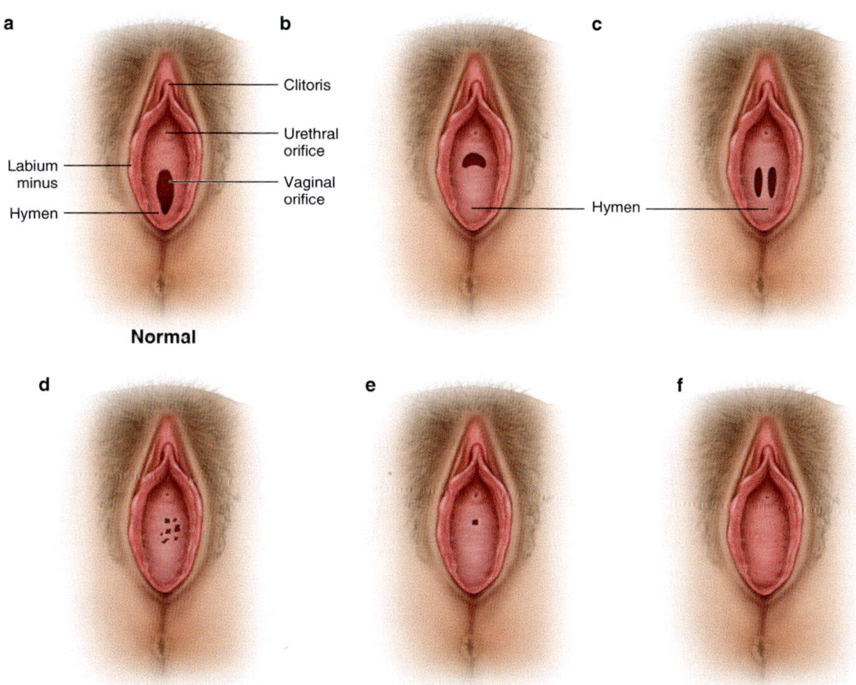

Fig. 1.4 Congenital anomalies of the hymen

1.2.2.2 Vagina Anomalies

Vaginal Agenesis

Vaginal agenesis is also known as MRKHs (Mayer-Rokitansky-Küster-Hauser) syndrome which includes congenital absence of the uterus and vagina. It is a kind of functional defect in the reproductive tract characterized by no reproductive ability. At present, the etiology is unclear. In animal models, it could be demonstrated that WNT4 gene suppresses male gonadal differentiation and ovarian androgen secretion; the absence of this gene might be related to this disorder [5].

Congenital vaginal agenesis is often accompanied by cervical or uterine abnormalities; 7–10 % of these patients have rudimentary uterine horn or cervical aplasia (Fig. 1.5), while the majorities have normal ovarian function. Seventy-eight percent of patients have normal uterus, 16 % with ovaries outside the pelvis, and 6 % with unilateral abnormal ovarian development [11]. These patients are often associated with other nongenital anomalies. Twenty-five to fifty percent of patients have urinary tract anomalies, including pelvic kidney or unilateral renal agenesis; 10–15 % also have skeletal anomalies mainly spinal deformities. Other rare anomalies include congenital heart disease, hand anomalies, deafness, cleft palate, and inguinal hernia.

Clinical manifestations are primary amenorrhea and sexual difficulties. Generally the patient has only a primitive uterus without periodic abdominal pain. Physical examination shows normal physical appearance, with normal secondary sexual characteristics and external genitalia, but there is no vaginal opening or only a shallow concave at the posterior part of vestibule. Occasionally there is a short vagina with a closed end.

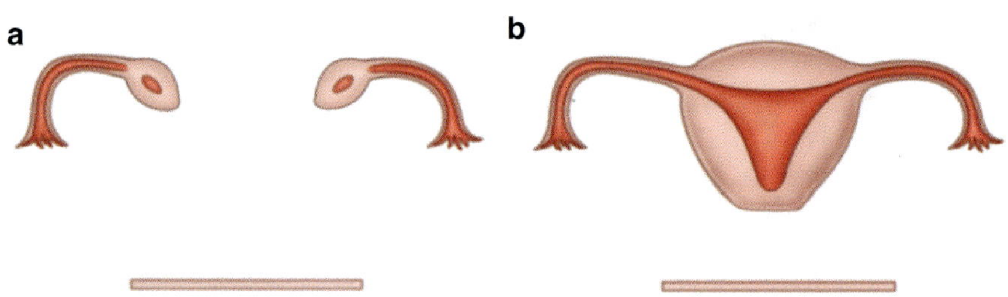

Fig. 1.5 Vaginal agenesis. (**a**) With rudimentary horns. (**b**) With cervical aplasia

Agenesis of the Lower Vagina

In the lower vaginal agenesis (Fig. 1.2 2), the upper vagina, cervix, and uterus are normal, but it is often associated with external genital anomalies. The clinical manifestations are primary amenorrhea, periodic abdominal pain, etc. Because the endometrium functions normally, these symptoms can occur early. Pelvic examination reveals a low-positioned pelvic mass, located in front of the rectum. Often treatment can be offered timely, because their symptoms present early similar to the imperforate hymen. On examination, there is no vaginal opening and the mucosal surface of the posterior vestibule shows normal color without any outward bulging. Digital rectal examination shows a palpable mass protruding into the rectum, but at a higher position than that in the imperforate hymen. It is also associated with lesser blood reflux into the peritoneal cavity causing pelvic endometriosis.

Transverse Vaginal Septum

It is caused by the failure to the fusion of the end the paramesonephric ducts which either do not open up or only partially open together with the urogenital sinus. The incidence rate is about 1/30,000 to 1/80,000 [7]. This condition is rarely associated with urinary tract and other organ abnormalities. The septum can be located in any part of the vagina; 46 % occurred at the upper part, 35–40 % at the middle, and 15–20 % at the lower part of the vagina. The septal thickness is usually less than 1 cm. If there is no hole in the septum, it is a complete transverse septum. If there are some small holes, it is an incomplete transverse septum (Figs. 1.2 (IIIB2) and 1.6). Transverse vaginal septum at the upper end of the vagina is often an incomplete septum, while the one at the lower end is often a complete septum.

Incomplete transverse septa at the upper vagina are often asymptomatic, while those at lower positions can affect sex life and also affect the descent of fetal presenting part at vaginal delivery. A patient with complete septum will present with primary amenorrhea and periodic abdominal pain which is progressively severe. Vaginal gynecological examination reveals a short vagina with a blind end or with a small pore across the center of the septum. On rectal examination, the cervix and uterus are palpable. Because a complete septum causes retention of menstrual blood, a mass can be palpable above the septum.

Transverse vaginal septum, at various positions of the vagina, can be a complete or incomplete transverse vaginal septum.

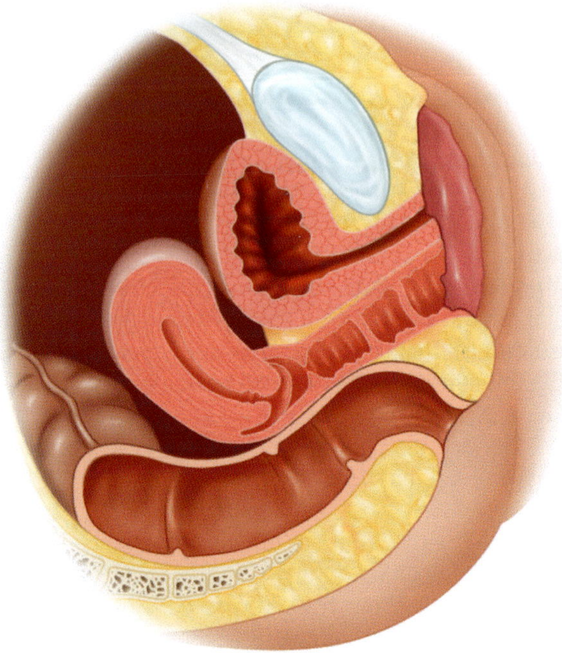

Fig. 1.6 Transverse vaginal septum

Longitudinal Vaginal Septum

It is caused by the partial fusion failure of the paramesonephric ducts with the lower ends of their wall persisted or only partially disappeared. They can be either a complete or an incomplete longitudinal septum. As a result, the vagina is divided into two longitudinal tunnels lined by mucosal wall and separated by a septum. A complete longitudinal septum extends from the cervix at the top and down to the vaginal opening at the lower end. An incomplete septum extends from the top, but does not reach the vaginal opening. A complete septum is often associated with a didelphic uterus, double cervices, and underdevelopment of a kidney on one side.

A complete longitudinal vaginal septum is often asymptomatic, with no impact on sex life and vaginal delivery. An incomplete longitudinal septum may have sex problems or discomfort. During labor, the descent of the fetal presenting part can be obstructed by the septum. Vaginal examination can reveal a longitudinal vaginal septum dividing the vagina into two longitudinal tunnels, with the top end of the septal mucosal wall close to the cervix, and for a complete longitudinal septum, the lower part of the septum reaches the vaginal opening, while for the incomplete longitudinal septum, it fails to reach the vaginal opening.

Oblique Vaginal Septum

The etiology is yet unclear and it may be that the paramesonephric ducts in the process extending downward do not reach the urogenital sinus and form a dead end. Oblique vaginal septum is often accompanied by ipsilateral urinary tract anomalies, often presenting with uterus didelphys, double cervices, and ipsilateral renal agenesis.

There are three types of oblique vaginal septum (Fig. 1.7).

Type I: Oblique septum without holes. The uterus behind the septum is completely separated from the uterus on the other side and also with the outside. The menstrual blood accumulates in the uterine cavity and the vaginal cavity behind the septum.

Type II: Oblique septum with a hole. The hole is a few millimeters in size. The uterus behind the septum is completely separated from the uterus on the other side. The menstrual blood can be discharged through the hole, but with poor drainage.

Type III: Oblique septum without holes combined with a cervical fistula. There is a small fistula between the two adjacent cervices or between a cervix and the adjacent vaginal cavity behind the septum on the other side. The menstrual blood in the uterine cavity on the side of the septum can be discharged via the small fistula to the cervix on the other side, but it is also with poor drainage.

In younger patients, their menstrual periods are regular and normal. All three types of vaginal septum will present with dysmenorrhea. Type I has more severe dysmenorrhea, usually with lower abdominal pain on one side. Type II has a small amount of vaginal discharge or intermenstrual brownish spotting or even smelly purulent discharge. Type III has prolonged menstrual period with spotting, but also may have purulent discharge. Gynecological examination of the side of the closed vaginal end may show a cystic tumor. For type I, the mass is harder and the retained uterine blood can lead to an enlarged uterus. For type II and III, the cystic masses are less distended, and old blood can flow out when pressed.

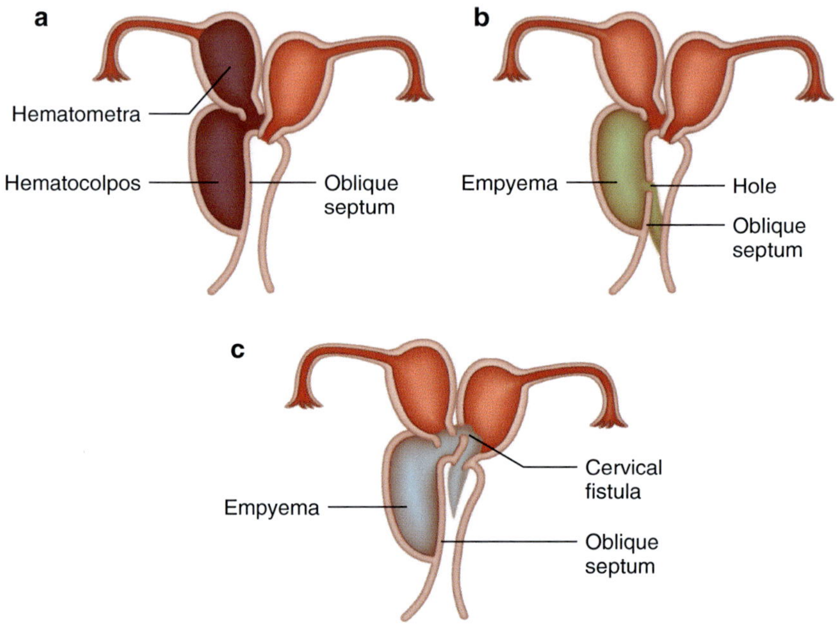

Fig. 1.7 Three types of oblique vaginal septum. (**a**) Septum without holes. (**b**) Septum with a hole. (**c**) Oblique septum without holes, but with a cervical fistula

Fig. 1.8 Congenital cervical anomalies. (**a**) Cervical agenesis; (**b**) cervical hypoplasia; (**c**) double cervices, double vaginas and bicornuate uterus; (**d**) septate uterus and longitudinal septa of cervix and vagina; (**e**) double cervices, double vaginas and complete septate uterus; (**f**) double cervices, double vaginas and single uterus; (**g**) septate cervix with double uteri; (**h**) double cervices, double vaginas, double uteri with low fistula; (**i**) as in H with type III oblique vaginal septum; (**j**) double cervices, double vaginas, incomplete septate uterus; (**k**) cervical septum with longitudinal vaginal septum and incomplete septate uterus

1.2.2.3 Cervical Aplasia or Hypoplasia

The new hypothesis is that the cervix is developed at about the 10th week of gestation. At the time of fusion, the lower ends of both Müllerian ducts fuse with the urogenital sinus isthmus beginning at the cervix. After the completion of Müllerian ducts fusion, reabsorption of the septum between both Müllerian ducts will form the body of the uterus with the upper segment of the cervix forming the internal os and the lower end forming the external os. Fusion and subsequent reabsorption progress toward the tip and tail of the fused Müllerian tubercle, while the tail end of the Müllerian tubercle forms the vagina. Both upper and lower ends of the Müllerian ducts fuse and reabsorb at different points in time. Any error in the development will lead to cervical agenesis, hypoplasia, or double cervices, sometimes associated with various vaginal, uterine, and urinary anomalies. Isolated cervical agenesis or hypoplasia is rare. The cervical agenesis is usually associated with upper vaginal anomaly, while cervical hypoplasia can have a normal vagina. Double cervices and cervical septum can be difficult to distinguish from their external appearance, and they are asymptomatic when there is no outflow obstruction. Some rare cervical anomalies cannot fall in line with the recommended American Society for Reproductive Medicine classification system of female reproductive tract anomalies (Fig. 1.8).

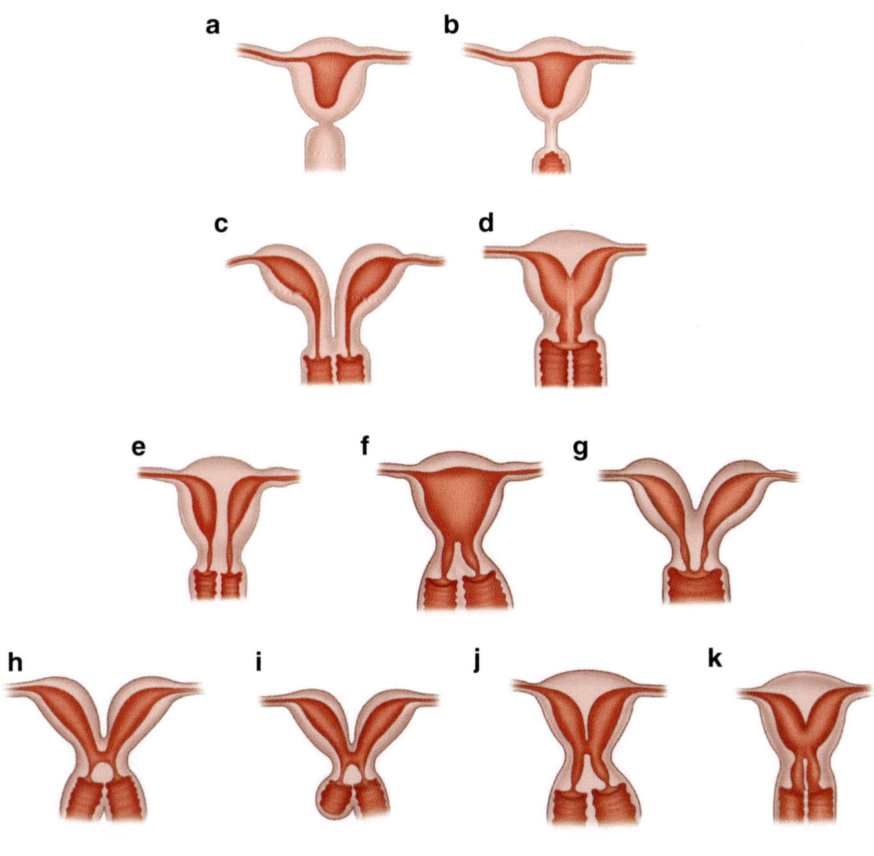

1.2.2.4 Uterine Anomalies

Congenital uterine anomalies often do not present with any symptoms and not being noticed. Therefore, it is difficult to determine its exact incidence. In women with normal childbirth, 2–4 % may be associated with uterine anomalies. The most common anomalies are uterine septum (90 %), double uterine horns (5 %), and double uteri (5 %). For women with adverse obstetrical history and recurrent miscarriages, the incidence of uterine anomalies is 10–25 % [8]. In the general population, the incidences of various uterine anomalies are [9] septate uterus (35 %), double uterine horns (26 %), arcuate uterus (18 %), single uterine horn (10 %), double uteri (8 %), and uterine agenesis (3 %).

Uterine Agenesis or Uterine Hypoplasia

The cause is due to the failure of fusion and reabsorption at the uterine end of both paramesonephric ducts. It is often associated with absence of the vagina as described previously as the MRKH syndrome.

Unilateral Uterine Anomalies

It is usually due to abnormal Müllerian duct development, which results in the following common uterine anomalies:

Septate Uterus and Arcuate Uterus

Septate uterus has a normal uterine shape, but with two uterine cavities (Figs. 1.1 C4, C5, and 1.2 III-A5). A septate uterus is a result of failure to reabsorb the longitudinal uterine septum after the fusion of the paramesonephric ducts. There are two types of septate uterus: (1) complete septate uterus, the longitudinal septum extends from the fundus of the uterus to the internal cervical os, and (2) incomplete septate uterus, the longitudinal septum extends to a level above the internal cervical os. Usually they are asymptomatic.

Arcuate uterus (Fig. 1.2 III-A6) is due to the abnormal development at the fundus of the uterus. There is a depression in the middle of the uterine fundus with the uterine wall slightly protruding into the uterine cavity. It is usually asymptomatic. On examination, there is a palpable depression at the fundus of the uterus which may suggest an arcuate uterus. The clinical manifestations of an arcuate uterus are their possible impacts on the pregnancy outcome; these include recurrent miscarriages, premature delivery, and premature rupture of membranes. But these are still controversial [10]. Among patients with adverse pregnancy outcomes, there are 21–44 % spontaneous abortions, 12–33 % premature delivery, and the remaining 50–72 % normal delivery.

Unicornuate Uterus

Only one of the paramesonephric ducts develops normally, forming a single uterine horn (Figs. 1.1b, 1.2 III-A2 and 1.3 U4), with a normal functioning ipsilateral ovary. The other paramesonephric duct becomes agenesis, tubular, or hypoplasia, with an undeveloped ovary. Both the fallopian tube and kidney on the same side are often absent. A part of the paramesonephric duct may form a rudimentary uterine horn. Single uterine horn has an incidence of 1: 4020, particularly higher in infertile women. Approximately 65 % of single uterine horn is associated with rudimentary uterine horn. The rudimentary uterine horn may be with or without a uterine cavity which may or may not connect with the single uterine horn. Forty percent of the single uterine horn is associated with renal abnormality. This anomaly is often related to some obstetric complications, e.g., ectopic pregnancy 2.7 %, early trimester miscarriage 24.3 %, mid-trimester miscarriage 9.7 %, premature birth 20.1 %, and intrauterine fetal death 10.5 %. Only 49.9 % of these patients can have live births [11].

A unicornuate uterus is asymptomatic. If its associated rudimentary uterine horn has functional endometrium and its cavity does not communicate with that of the unicornuate uterus, this will lead to retrograde blood flow into the pelvic cavity, and this can cause dysmenorrhea and pelvic endometriosis. Vaginal examination may show a small, spindle-shaped unicornuate uterus deviated from the midline. If it is accompanied by a rudimentary horn, a smaller lump can be palpable next to the uterus. This may be misdiagnosed as an ovarian cyst or tumor. If there is menstrual bleeding inside the cavity of the rudimentary horn, a tender lump can be palpable due to a uterine hematoma.

Bicornuate Uterus

Bicornuate uterus has a significant depression at the fundus with its appearance quite different from a septate uterus (Figs. 1.1 C7, C8, and 1.2 III-A4). It is due to a failure of the fusion of bilateral paramesonephric ducts. Depending the separation of uterine cavity, it can be a complete double uterus (separation begins from the internal cervical os) or an incomplete double uterus (separation from above the internal cervical os) and the arcuate uterus (this latter is in dispute). Patients usually do not have any clinical symptom. But sometimes there can be heavy menstrual bleeding, associated with various degrees of dysmenorrhea. On examination, a depression can be palpable at the fundus of the uterus.

Didelphic Uterus

Didelphic uterus is formed when both paramesonephric ducts did not fuse together, and they separately develop into two uteri and two cervices. The two cervices can be separated or connected with a communicating fistula. Most didelphic uteri have favorable pregnancy outcome. However, one of the cervices may not develop normally or even absent, but there may be a small fistula connecting it with the adjacent vagina. A didelphic uterus can be associated with a longitudinal vaginal septum or an oblique septum, but patients usually do not have any symptoms if there is no outflow obstruction.

Abnormal Vertical Fusion of the Uterus

Abnormal Müllerian ducts fusion with the urogenital tubercle or abnormal vaginal recanalization will lead to cervical agenesis, hypoplasia, or vaginal septum.

Diethylstilbestrol-Related Uterine Anomalies

Diethylstilbestrol, a synthetic estrogen, had been used from 1949 to 1971. The in vivo exposure to diethylstilbestrol can cause developmental defects of the paramesonephric ducts associated with various fetal malformations, including (1) female fetus that can have uterine anomalies like a small T-shaped uterine cavity, a narrow uterine cavity, or a uterus with widened lower uterine segment and irregular uterine wall (the T- shaped uterine cavity is the most common diethylstilbestrol-related uterine anomaly (42–62 %)); (2) vaginal adenosis, vaginal ridges, and transverse vaginal septum; and (3) cervical anomalies with hypoplasia.

1.2.2.5 Fallopian Tubes Anomalies

Tubal developmental abnormality is rare. It is caused by developmental blockage at the top end of the paramesonephric ducts, and it often coexists with uterine anomalies. Almost all are discovered incidentally at surgery because of other diseases.

Absence or Remnant of Fallopian Tubes

The absence and remnant of the fallopian tube is the result of an undeveloped ipsilateral paramesonephric duct, often accompanied with ipsilateral abnormal development of the ureter and kidney. There is yet no reported case of a simple absence of both fallopian tubes. Absence of fallopian tube is often accompanied with severe abnormalities of other internal organs, and as such the fetus cannot survive.

Abnormal Development of Fallopian Tubes

It is a common genital anomaly. The fallopian tubes can be small, slender, and curving, with various degree of abnormal tubal wall development, tubes without lumen, and partly obliterated lumen. All these can result in infertility. Tubal diverticulum or abnormal tubal orifice can be a cause of ectopic pregnancy.

Supernumerary Fallopian Tube(s)

Attaching to one or both of the fallopian tubes, there is another smaller tube with fimbrial end. In some cases, there is a communication between the normal fallopian tube and this smaller tube and some do not.

Supernumerary Normal Fallopian Tube(s)

There is/are normally developed fallopian tube(s) either unilateral or bilateral. They are all communicated with the uterine cavity.

1.2.2.6 Ovarian Anomalies

Ovarian anomaly is due to the blockage of primordial germ cell migration or the abnormal shift in location at the formation of gonads.

Ovarian Agenesis or Ovarian Anomalies

Unilateral or bilateral agenesis of ovaries is extremely rare. Unilateral or bilateral hypoplastic ovaries are white in appearance, as slender cords. They are also known as streak ovaries. Sectioning of a hypoplastic ovary shows only fibrous tissue without follicles. The clinical manifestations include primary amenorrhea or delayed menarche, scanty menstruation, and poor secondary sexual characteristics. It is often accompanied by abnormal development of genital or urinary organs and more commonly seen in patients with Turner's syndrome.

Ectopic Ovaries

After the formation of ovaries, they remain in the primitive genital ridge area, without descent to the pelvis. Patients with ectopic ovaries have normal ovarian functions and are asymptomatic.

Supernumerary Ovaries

The supernumerary ovary is rare. It is generally far away from the normal position of the ovary and in a retroperitoneal position. It is asymptomatic and more often found incidentally during surgery for other diseases.

References

1. The American Fertility Society classifications of adnexal adhesions, distal tubal occlusion, tubal occlusion secondary to tubal ligation, tubal pregnancies, Mullerian anomalies and intrauterine adhesions[J]. Fertil Steril. 1988;49:944–55.
2. Minto CL, Hollings N, Hall-Craggs M, et al. Magnetic resonance imaging in the assessment of complex Mullerian anomalies[J]. BJOG: Int J Obstet Gynaecol. 2001;108:791–7.
3. Acien P, Acien MI. The history of female genital tract malformation classifications and proposal of an updated system[J]. Hum Reprod Update. 2011;17:693–705.

4. Grimbizis GF, Gordts S, Di Spiezio SA, et al. The ESHRE/ESGE consensus on the classification of female genital tract congenital anomalies[J]. Hum Reprod. 2013;28:2032–44.
5. Biason-Lauber A, Konrad D, Navratil F, et al. A WNT4 mutation associated with Mullerian-duct regression and virilization in a 46, XX woman[J]. N Engl J Med. 2004;351:792–8.
6. Fedele L, Bianchi S, Frontino G, et al. Laparoscopic findings and pelvic anatomy in Mayer-Rokitansky-Kuster-Hauser syndrome[J]. Obstet Gynecol. 2007;109:1111–5.
7. Rock JA, Azziz R. Genital anomalies in childhood[J]. Clin Obstet Gynecol. 1987;30:682–96.
8. Acien P. Incidence of Mullerian defects in fertile and infertile women[J]. Hum Reprod. 1997;12:1372–6.
9. Grimbizis GF, Camus M, Tarlatzis BC, et al. Clinical implications of uterine malformations and hysteroscopic treatment results[J]. Hum Reprod Update. 2001;7:161–74.
10. Heinonen PK. Complete septate uterus with longitudinal vaginal septum[J]. Fertil Steril. 2006;85:700–5.
11. Reichman D, Laufer MR, Robinson BK. Pregnancy outcomes in unicornuate uteri: a review[J]. Fertil Steril. 2009;91:1886–94.

Chapter 2
The Diagnosis of Female Reproductive Tract Anomalies

Xiaochuan Li, Lan Zhu, Qing Dai, and Jingjing Lu

2.1 Introduction

Xiaochuan Li and Lan Zhu

Female genital anomalies are mainly referred to the female reproductive tract abnormalities or abnormal gonad development with or without other organ malformations. It is a large class of abnormal developmental diseases involving the vulva, vagina, uterus, fallopian tubes, and ovaries.

Female genital anomalies are based mainly on their clinical symptoms, physical examinations, and basic imaging studies to make a preliminary diagnosis, further assisted by chromosomal analysis, hormone assessment, diagnostic imaging, and even diagnostic surgical procedure to obtain an accurate diagnosis. The common clinical manifestations of these diseases are as follows:

Primary amenorrhea: It is the clinical symptoms ion women over 14 years of age who do not have any menstruation and secondary sexual characteristics or over 16 years of age when they have secondary sexual characteristics but without menstruation. About 50 % of the patients with primary amenorrhea are due to gonadal anomalies and 20 % due for reproductive tract abnormalities such as congenital absence of vagina, imperforate hymen, etc.

X. Li • L. Zhu (✉)
Department of Obstetrics and Gynecology, Peking Union Medical College Hospital,
No. 1 Shuaifuyuan, Beiijing 100730, P. R. China
e-mail: zhu_julie@sina.com

Q. Dai
Department of Ultrasound, Peking Union Medical College Hospital,
No. 1 Shuaifuyuan, Beijing 100730, P. R. China

J. Lu
Department of Radiology, Peking Union Medical College Hospital,
No. 1 Shuaifuyuan, Beiijing 100730, P. R. China

© Springer Science+Business Media Dordrecht 2015

L. Zhu et al. (eds.), *Atlas of Surgical Correction of Female Genital Malformation*,
DOI 10.1007/978-94-017-7246-4_2

Symptoms related to reproductive tract obstruction: the most common symptoms are dysmenorrhea and periodic lower abdominal pain. These symptoms are often due to the presence of functional endometrium, and the menstrual outflow is obstructed. Because of retrograde menstruation, some patients present with endometriosis-related disorders of the ovaries, uterus, and pelvic endometriosis. When the menstrual outflow is incompletely obstructed, there will be irregular menstrual spotting with poor menstrual flow. When the obstruction is associated with infection, pus can form in the vagina or uterine cavity presenting as acute pelvic inflammatory disease. Obstruction at the vagina will have typical cyclical abdominal pain with increasing severity; symptoms due to imperforate hymen, transverse vaginal septum, and vaginal oblique septum may vary depending whether there are holes in the septum or not, causing either complete or incomplete obstruction symptoms.

The impact on pregnancy and delivery outcome: Different types of uterine anomalies may be related to miscarriage, premature birth, fetal malposition, fetal growth retardation, abnormal progress of labor, and postpartum hemorrhage. Rudimentary uterine horn pregnancy can lead to life-threatening uterine rupture. Among female patients with infertility, 10 % are associated with anomalies of the vulva, vagina, cervix, or uterus.

Sexual difficulties: It is common for patients with genital anomalies to complain of sexual difficulties, but rarely as the only symptom. There are usually complaints together with symptoms related to reproductive tract obstruction.

Ambiguous sexual genitalia or external genital abnormalities: Abnormal gonadal differentiation (true hermaphroditism, gonadal dysgenesis, etc.), androgen excess (congenital adrenal hyperplasia, excessive exogenous androgen exposure in early pregnancy, etc.), androgen deficiency (partial androgen insensitivity syndrome, testicular regression syndrome, etc.), and genitourinary tubercle anomalies (persistent cloaca, labia minora fusion, etc.) can cause this clinical manifestation. Ambiguous sexual genitalia can be combined with the internal genital anomalies, urinary tract anomalies, and/or anorectal malformation. Serious ambiguous sexual genitalia are more commonly found and corrected in the neonatal or infantile period, but improper corrective treatment or atypical symptoms will make it difficult for the diagnosis and subsequent treatment in the future.

The symptoms of urinary tract anomalies: 30–50 % of patients with genital anomalies are associated with urinary tract anomalies. The majority of the urinary tract anomalies are asymptomatic, yet some may present with symptoms of urinary tract infection, hematuria, urinary frequency, urgency, dysuria, and so on. Patients with urogenital fistula like vesicovaginal fistula may present with menstrual hematuria. Some patients with urogenital sinus malformation may have abnormally slack urethral opening that may be mistaken as the vaginal opening. They will present with painful sexual intercourse, sexual difficulties, stress urinary incontinence, and recurrent urinary tract infections.

Related symptoms of other organ malformations: Female genital anomalies are often associated with other organ malformations. Attention should be paid to the height, skeletal abnormalities, deafness, and other deformities of these patients.

Asymptomatic: A study of female genital anomalies among patients who had had tubal ligation showed that 3.2 % of those asymptomatic females had Müllerian duct anomalies. Therefore, some scholars estimated that the incidence of the female genital anomalies could be as high as 7 % in the general population and the majority of them were asymptomatic.

When patients presented with the above clinical manifestations, they should be included in the "high-risk" group for female genital anomalies. Progressive investigations start from different levels, from simple to complex, and from noninvasive to invasive; careful inspection and evaluation of complaints will help to raise the clinical awareness and lead to the diagnosis of these disorders. Other assessments should include detailed medical history and physical examination, sex chromosome analysis, gonadal hormone levels, and imaging assessment and finally with diagnostic surgery if it is necessary.

2.1.1 *Medical History and Physical Examination*

Medical history includes mother's pregnancy history and family history: whether there was any drug exposure that occurred during pregnancy, whether there were chemicals from the environment which interfered endocrine secretions, whether there had been diethylstilbestrol (DES) exposure in early pregnancy, and so on. Family history includes other family members (especially sisters) who might have similar clinical symptoms or known genital anomalies and have suffered early neonatal death and inbreeding childbearing and other family members (especially aunts) with infertility, amenorrhea, premature menopause, and so on. Despite the causes for the majority of female genital anomalies need to be further elucidated, but at least there is familial aggregation of these diseases or there are certainly genetic characteristics, it clearly has made them genetic-related diseases.

In physical examination, the keys to make a diagnosis are the number of gonads and their positions whether they are abnormal and the certainty of the anatomy of the reproductive tract. Other examinations are to identify the other characteristic features of malformation syndromes, such as Turner syndrome (congenital ovarian hypoplasia). The typical characteristics of Turner syndrome are short stature (usually less than 150 cm), epicanthus, webbed neck, and elbow valgus. It is therefore important to familiarize with these phenotypic characteristics that will facilitate the diagnosis of genetic-related genital anomalies.

2.1.2 Sex Chromosome Analysis

Reproductive tract development and sexual differentiation are closely related to the sex chromosomes which are the basis for the gender differentiation which is one of the most critical steps of sex differentiation. Sex chromosome analysis helps to contribute to the diagnosis and differential diagnosis of female genital anomalies. Common chromosomal abnormalities causing genital anomalies are as follows: (1) Turner syndrome (congenital ovarian hypoplasia) chromosome 45, XO, expressed as ovarian dysgenesis and juvenile external and internal genitalia, accompanied with multiple organs malformations and (2) triple X chromosome 47, XXX, expressed as female phenotype but poorly developed breasts and genitalia with ovarian atrophy. Some patients may have menstrual cycles, secondary amenorrhea, and premature menopause. There is often mentally retardation. Chromosome analysis also helps to distinguish true hermaphroditism, XO/XY gonadal dysgenesis, and the like. However, in many patients with female genital anomalies, their chromosome analysis usually shows normal female phenotype.

2.1.3 Gonadal and Sex Hormone Assessment

After the sex chromosomes determine the gender, gonadal differentiation and development would lead to the differentiation and development of internal and external genitalia. The final phenotypic sex will finally develop under the influence of sex hormones. When there is gonadal dysgenesis or abnormal sex hormone synthesis or dysfunction, it could lead to genital anomalies. By measuring the serum sex hormones and gonadotropin, it helps to make the diagnosis. For example, in patients with 46, XX pure gonadal dysgenesis, their chromosome analysis and external appearance are all phenotypic female, yet they cannot develop secondary sexual characteristics. The laboratory tests will show a low serum estrogen and increased serum gonadotropin. The clinical presentation will be primary amenorrhea. Another example is the congenital adrenal hyperplasia. The chromosome karyotype is 46, XX, but it is the abnormal synthesis of cortisol that caused by the deficiency of an adrenal enzyme, leading to increased adrenal steroid precursors to generate excessive androgens. High serum 17α-hydroxyprogesterone, high testosterone, and positive dexamethasone suppression test can confirm the diagnosis.

2.1.4 Imaging Examination

Commonly used imaging examinations include ultrasound imaging, X-ray, MRI, CT scan, hysterosalpingography (HSG), and so on. The main aims of imaging are (1) to indicate the site of anomaly, anatomical features, and any related complication and (2) to exclude any morphological abnormalities in other organs. Ultrasound imaging is most widely used as a preliminary investigation because it is noninvasive, simple, and economical. MRI has an advantage in the examinations of cervix, uterine, and complicated pelvic abnormalities. It is often used as a confirmative diagnostic test. X-ray and CT scan are valuable methods for investigating skeletal malformations, but they are inferior to MRI and ultrasound for the diagnosis of female genital anomalies. HSG is useful to determine the size and shape of the uterine cavity, but because it is invasive with ionizing radiation, it is gradually replaced by ultrasound and MRI examination.

2.1.5 Diagnostic Surgical Procedures

If a certain diagnosis cannot be made despite all of the above investigations and examinations, or if there are indications for surgical treatment for the patients, diagnostic (treatment) surgery may be used as the last resort. Hysteroscopy, laparoscopy, or sometimes a combination of both is used. During a diagnostic procedure, pathological examination may be helpful for the final diagnosis. Sometimes a therapeutic surgical treatment if indicated can be completed simultaneously.

2.2 Ultrasound Diagnosis of Female Genital Anomalies

Qing Dai

During the embryonic development of female genital organs, there are internal or external influences which can lead to genital anomalies. The common reproductive tract anomalies are (1) vulvar anomalies, e.g., the imperforate hymen; (2) vaginal anomalies, e.g., congenital absence of vagina, vaginal atresia, transverse vaginal septum, longitudinal vaginal septum, and oblique vaginal septum; and (3) uterine anomalies, e.g., congenital absence of uterus, primordial uterus, infantile uterus, uterus didelphys, bicornuate uterus, rudimentary horn, arcuate uterus, septate uterus, and so on.

Imaging examination plays a very important role in the diagnosis of female reproductive tract anomalies. The commonly used imaging methods include ultrasound, X-ray imaging, MRI, CT scan, etc., in which ultrasound is the most commonly chosen method.

2.2.1 Ultrasound Imaging

Ultrasound imaging has been used in clinical obstetrics and gynecology for nearly half a century. With the ongoing development of ultrasound equipment, the image quality of ultrasound scan has greatly improved. It now plays an increasingly important role in the diagnosis and management of reproductive tract anomalies. Many uterine anomalies can also be discovered by ultrasound imaging examination alone.

Ultrasound examination techniques are as follows.

2.2.1.1 Abdominal Ultrasonography

Abdominal ultrasound examination involves placing an ultrasonic transducer on the abdominal wall for scanning. It is the most common imaging examination, suitable for all women requiring pelvic ultrasound examination.

1. Before abdominal ultrasound examination, the patient has to drink 500–1000 ml of water to fill the bladder before the test.
2. The patient has to lie in a conventional supine position for examination.
3. An ultrasonic transducer with a convex array probe at a frequency of 3.5–5.0 MHz should be used.
4. Ultrasound gel is applied to the exposed lower abdomen and ultrasound scanning probe is applied directly on the skin.
5. The scanning method is to conduct a longitudinal section scanning, and then rotate the probe 90° to observe the transverse section image. Based on the lesion or regions of interest, the probe is moved flexibly and the scanning direction and angle are changed for oblique surface scanning if necessary, in order to obtain the best image of the lesion and the region of interest.

2.2.1.2 Transvaginal Ultrasonography

Transvaginal ultrasound examination involves placing the vaginal ultrasound probe for the examination. As the probe is closer to the pelvic organs at this time, it can display clearly any mass associated with the uterus, ovaries, and pelvis.

1. The patient has to empty the bladder before the scan examination.
2. The patient has to lie supine in a lithotomy position.
3. A vaginal probe with probe frequency of 5.0–7.5 MHz is used.
4. A disposable latex condom is used covering the tip of the vaginal probe before the application of the coupling ultrasound jelly; operator holds the vaginal probe with the right hand and puts the probe slowly into the vagina until the top of the probe reaches the vaginal fornix.
5. During scanning, use rotation, tilt, pumping, and other basic techniques to conduct longitudinal, coronal, and transverse section scanning for all the pelvic structures.

2.2.1.3 Transrectal Ultrasonography

Transrectal ultrasound examination involves placing a rectal or vaginal ultrasound probe (now the majority of ultrasound equipment use the same probe) into the rectum for scanning. This scan is more often used for ultrasound examination of the male prostate. Uses in gynecology are mainly for those when abdominal scans are not clear and transvaginal ultrasound cannot be used in children and unmarried women, women with severe vaginal atrophy, etc. Before the examination, patient must empty their stool and urine, generally on the previous night by taking laxatives. During the scan, patient has to take a left lateral position or lie supine in a lithotomy position. A latex condom is used to cover the probe tip, and after the application of coupling ultrasound jelly over the head of the probe, it is then slowly inserted into the rectum. The scanning method is similar to that for a transvaginal scanning.

2.2.1.4 Perineal Ultrasonography

Perineal ultrasound examination involves placing the probe on the perineal area above the anus for scanning. Patients have to take a lithotomy position, with the probe head covered by a latex condom. The probe is placed in the area between the upper edge of the anus and the labia or on the surface of the labia majora at the vulva, for longitudinal and oblique coronal section scanning. When observing uterine adnexa, a convex array probe at frequency 3.5–5.0 MHz is used; when observing the vagina, a high-frequency linear transducer probe at frequency 5.0–12.0 MHz is used.

2.2.1.5 Ultrasound Saline Hysterography

Ultrasound saline hysterography is an ultrasound imaging method to examine the uterine cavity and other structures after the infusion of saline into the uterine cavity. An ultrasound imaging catheter (alternatives include urinary catheter, pediatric gastric tube, etc.) is inserted into the uterine cavity through the vagina and the cervix, and an appropriate amount of sterile saline is infused and fills up uterine cavity before conducting an abdominal or transvaginal ultrasound examination. For transvaginal examination, the patient has to lie supine in a lithotomy position with the probe placed in the vagina. Whether or not to use a three-way catheter with a saline distended catheter balloon at the catheter tip will depend on the tightness of the opening of the cervix and the ability to retain the saline in the uterine cavity. For ultrasound imaging, the non-echogenic saline in the uterine cavity creates good contrast with the medium to high echo signals of the endometrium. It permits an accurate evaluation of the endometrium and the uterine cavity. This method can also be used to observe the structure of the vagina. At this point, patient can be asked to raise up her buttocks. The catheter can be relocated directly in the upper vagina. The imaging can now display opened the closed upper vagina wall and reveal any incomplete oblique or transverse vaginal septum.

2.2.1.6 Three-Dimensional (3D) Ultrasonography

Three-dimensional ultrasound examination involves using a three-dimensional volume probe to collect numerous images from a targeted organ and reconstruct these images to obtain a 3D image. The examination methods and approaches are the same as the two-dimensional ultrasound. The difference is that three-dimensional ultrasonography must use a three-dimensional volume probe. When scanning, a three-dimensional volume probe is placed on the abdominal wall or inside the vagina (use an intravaginal volume probe), and scan the region required for examination. When the probe position is fixed, the 3D function can be started. Any adjustments to the three-dimensional sampling volume are made before the automatic volume scanning proceeds to obtain the 3D volume images. These images will be stored in the hard drive for analysis. Three-dimensional ultrasound imaging can be used to observe the coronal sections of reproductive organs, with the greater advantages in the diagnosis of congenital uterine abnormalities, such as septate uterus, uterus didelphys, bicornuate uterus, arcuate uterus, and so on.

Congenital uterine anomalies are the most common developmental abnormalities of the genital tract; hence it is of great clinical significance to learn these imaging features.

Congenital Absence of the Uterus

When the uterus is absent, it is because bilateral paramesonephric ducts stop growing medially to meet up at the midline. Its clinical manifestation is primary amenorrhea, but the secondary sexual characteristics are normal.

Ultrasound features: Both longitudinal scanning and transverse scanning of the lower abdomen do not detect the uterus behind the bladder.

Primordial Uterus

The bilateral paramesonephric ducts grow medially and meet up at the midline but then soon stopped growing. The resulting uterus is small and does not have uterine cavity or may have uterine cavity without endometrium. The clinical manifestation is primary amenorrhea.

Ultrasound features: The uterus is a small cord-like muscular structure with a diameter <2.0 cm, but it has no echo line to suggest a uterine cavity or no endometrial echo to suggest any endometrium (Fig. 2.1).

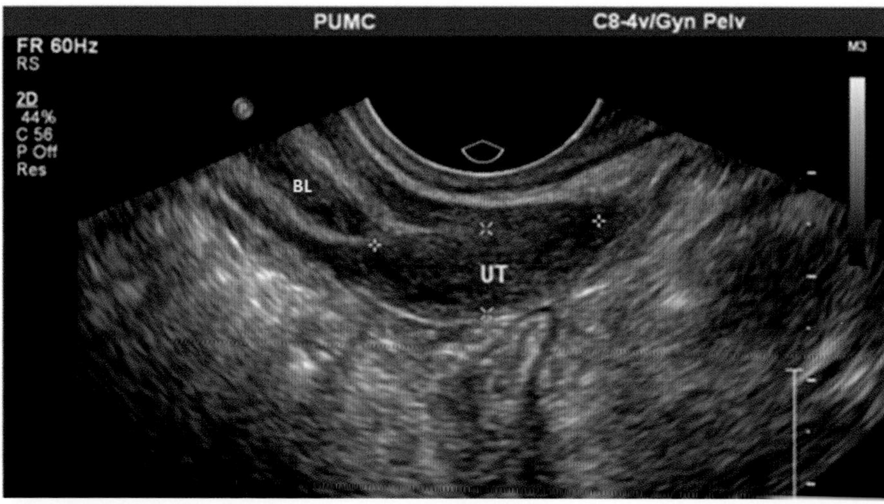

Fig. 2.1 A 23-year-old patient with primary amenorrhea. Transrectal ultrasonography showing a hypoechoic structure behind bladder *UT* and *BL*, with the size of 2.0×0.8 cm

Infantile Uterus

In late pregnancy or at any time from after birth to puberty, the uterus stops growing. After puberty, the ratio of the uterine body and the cervix is still the same at 1:2 as in infants and young children.

Ultrasound features: All uterine diameters are significantly smaller than a normal uterus; the anterior-posterior diameter (i.e., the thickness) is <2.0 cm; the cervix is relatively longer (Fig. 2.2).

Uterus Didelphys

Both bilateral paramesonephric ducts develop normally but do not join together at midline, so each side has a set of fallopian tube and uterus.

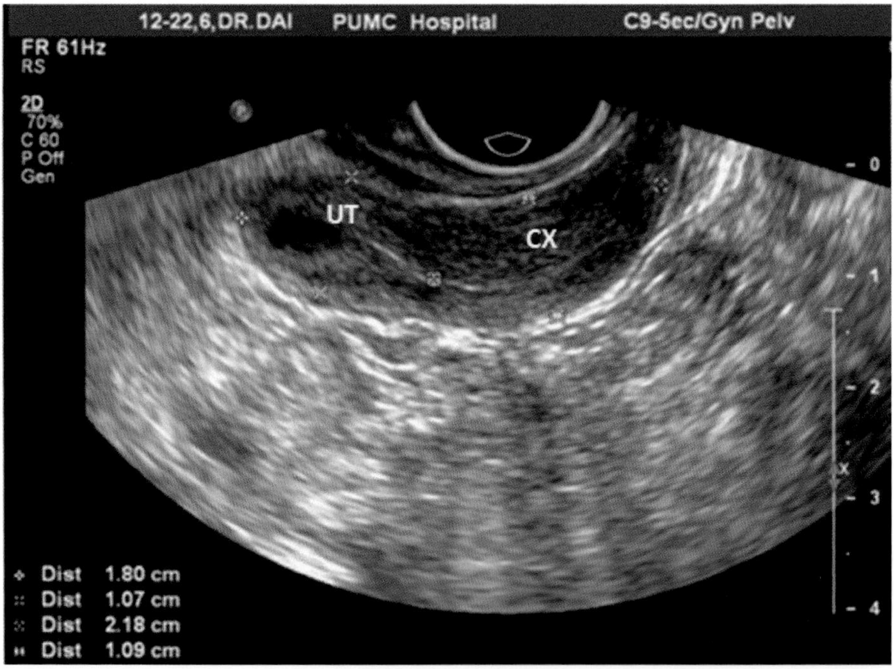

Fig. 2.2 Transvaginal ultrasound showing an infantile uterus. A 24-year-old patient presenting primary amenorrhea. All the uterine diameters are significantly smaller than normal with uterine body size: 1.8 × 1.5 × 1.1 cm, cervical length 2.2 cm, and body/cervix ratio <1

Ultrasound Features

Uterus didelphys under ultrasonic examination would show two completely separate uteri, which are particularly clear on coronal observation. The two completely separate uterine bodies have a deep depression in between them. Both show uterine endometrial echoes (Fig. 2.3); they may be associated with double cervix; then the cervical diameter can be seen widened with two cervical echoes next to each other but completely separated (Fig. 2.4a, b).

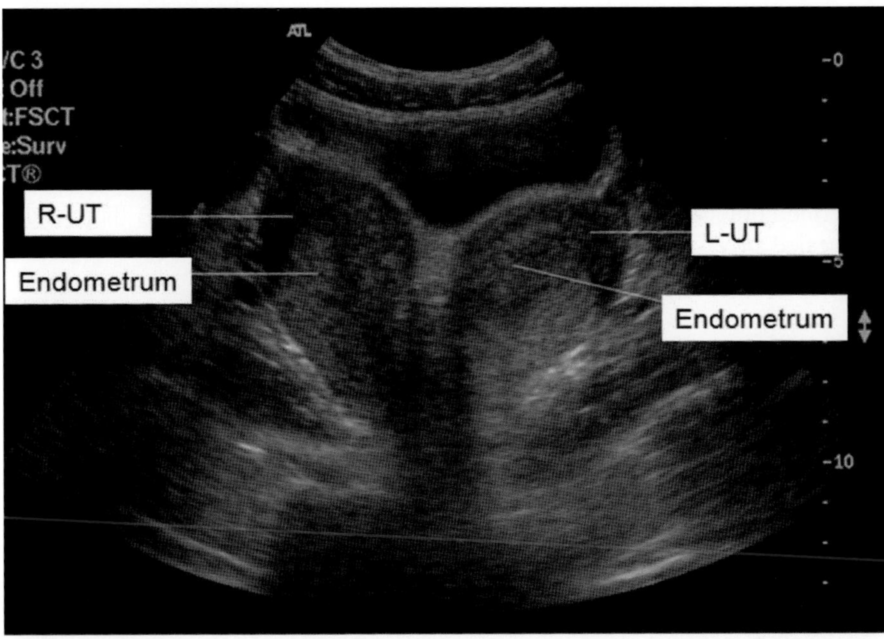

Fig. 2.3 Abdominal ultrasound showing double uterine abnormalities. It shows both the left and right uteri, with uterine body completely separated and two separate endometrial echoes

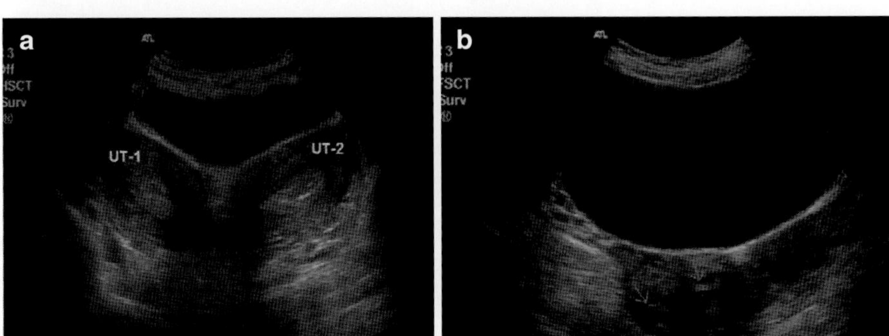

Fig. 2.4 Double uterine abnormalities (double uterus, double cervix): abdominal ultrasound showing cross-sectional images of two uteri and cervices. (**a**) Double uterus. (**b**) Double cervix

Bicornuate Uterus

The ends of the bilateral paramesonephric ducts joined, but not completely at the fundus of the uterus, resulting in a prominent horn on each side of the uterus.

Ultrasound Features

1. Two-dimensional ultrasonography: Bicornuate uterus should be best observed at cross-sectional scanning. The uterus can be seen with a widened fundus with a "saddle-shaped" depression at the middle (Fig. 2.5) or "Y"-shaped fundus; the uterine endometrial echo is also "Y" shaped.
2. Three-dimensional ultrasonography: Bicornuate uterus has two separate uterine horns; the upper uterine segment is completely separated but the lower uterine segment is still partly fused. Therefore, the three-dimensional ultrasonography of the coronal section directly shows a depression at the uterine fundus with two uterine horns as butterfly-shaped or as two leaves, and sometimes the bladder revealed a "V"-shaped pressure trace; the uterine endometrium is like a "butterfly wing."

Rudimentary Horn Uterus

The paramesonephric duct on one side developed normally, but the middle and lower segments of the contralateral paramesonephric duct have stopped growing, thus forming different degrees of rudimentary horn. According to presence or absence of endometrial cavity, it can be divided into either rudimentary horn with or without endometrium. The latter is further divided into either connected or not connected type of rudimentary horn according to whether its endometrial cavity is connected to the contralateral uterine cavity or not.

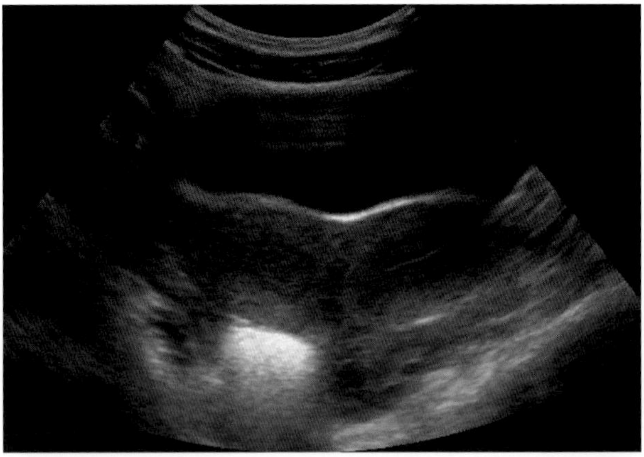

Fig. 2.5 Bicornuate uterus: an abdominal scan showing an abnormal uterine cross-sectional image, displaying a widened fundus with a saddle-shaped depression at the middle

The symptoms of rudimentary horn uterus pregnancy and interstitial tubal pregnancy are similar. They are asymptomatic in early pregnancy, but due to the poor muscular wall of the rudimentary horn, it cannot accommodate the growing fetus by becoming hypertrophied. The wall will break and rupture, usually from three to 4 months of pregnancy, thus causing severe bleeding and shock, threatening the life of the pregnant woman.

Ultrasound Features

1. Rudimentary horn may present as a normal uterus in the pelvis, but on one side, it shows a hypoechoic mass in which its echo is similar to that of the myometrium. It might look like a hypoechoic ribbon attached to the main body of the uterus (Fig. 2.6a, b). If it is not connected with the cervix, it can be easily confused as a subserous fibroid. A rudimentary uterine horn with uterine endometrium can be clearly visualized at the luteal phase of the menstrual cycle (Fig. 2.6c); if there are blood clots in the cavity, it may become an echo-free zone.

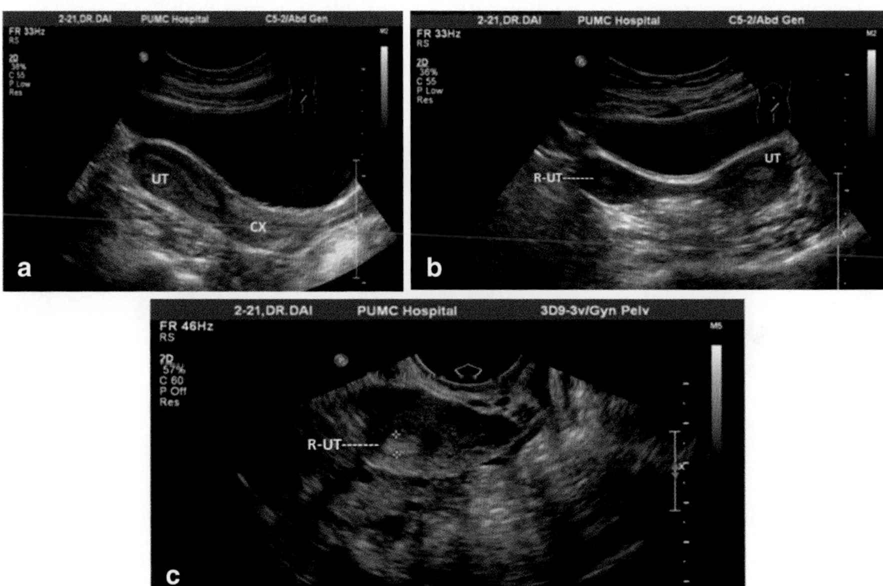

Fig. 2.6 Rudimentary uterine horn. (**a**) Abdominal ultrasound showing longitudinal uterine image. (**b**) Abdominal ultrasound showing a cross-sectional image of the uterus and rudimentary uterine horn with a hypoechoic ribbon connecting the horn with the main body of the uterus. (**c**) Transvaginal ultrasound showing rudimentary horn of the uterus and its endometrial echo (*UT* the body of the uterus palace, *CX* main uterine cervix, *R-UT* rudimentary horn of the uterus)

2. Rudimentary horn pregnancy: It is a round mass beside the normal uterus, in which a gestational sac could be seen. Around the gestational sac are obvious muscle tissues, but the endometrial layer around the gestational sac is not connected with the normal cervical canal. On the other hand, the normal uterus can have a thick decidual echo in its uterine cavity or the echo of a false gestational sac.

Septate Uterus

After the fusion of both paramesonephric ducts, the intervening septum has not been absorbed; this divides the uterine cavity into two halves within a normal uterus; if the septum is only partly absorbed, it is an incomplete septate uterus.

Ultrasound Features

1. Two-dimensional ultrasonography: The uterine appearance is normal, but the diameter of the uterine fundus is wider. Its cross-section shows two uterine endometrial echoes with a central echo of the septum (Fig. 2.7a, b). If the septum extends to the cervix, associated with two full endometrial echoes, it is a complete septate uterus; if the endometrial echoes from both sides merge in the middle or lower uterine cavity, it is an incomplete septate uterus.

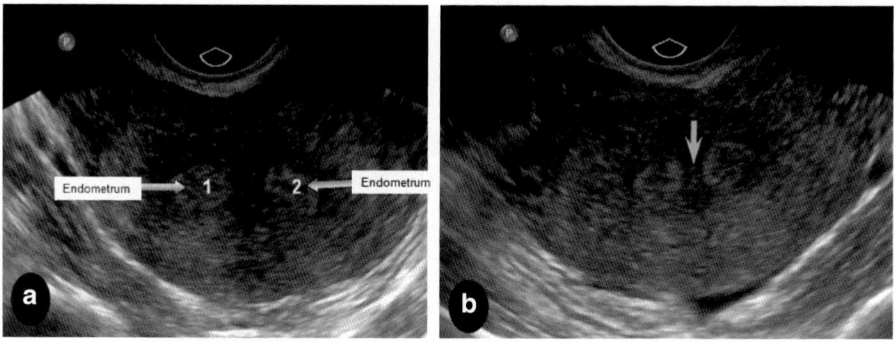

Fig. 2.7 Septate uterus: (**a**) an abdominal ultrasound showing a cross-sectional image of two endometrial echoes (marked by *arrows*) separated by a septum at the middle of the uterus. (**b**) A central septum (marked by an *arrow*) in the middle of the uterus

2. Three-dimensional ultrasonography: Two-dimensional ultrasound images are difficult to obtain a coronal imaging so it is more difficult to differentiate the types of septate uterus. Three-dimensional ultrasound scan can provide coronal uterine images, hence to obtain a direct visualization of the uterine endometrium. On a 3D coronal image, there is a clear low echo strip (septum) similar to the uterine muscular wall. The septum extends from the fundus of the uterus to the cervix, either reaching it (a complete septate uterus) or not reaching it (an incomplete septate uterus).

The two endometria of the incomplete septate uterus merge at the lower uterine segment at an acute angle <90° as a "Y"-shaped image (Fig. 2.8); for a complete septate uterus, the septum reaches the cervix, and the uterine endometria image present as a "V"-shaped image (Fig. 2.9a, b).

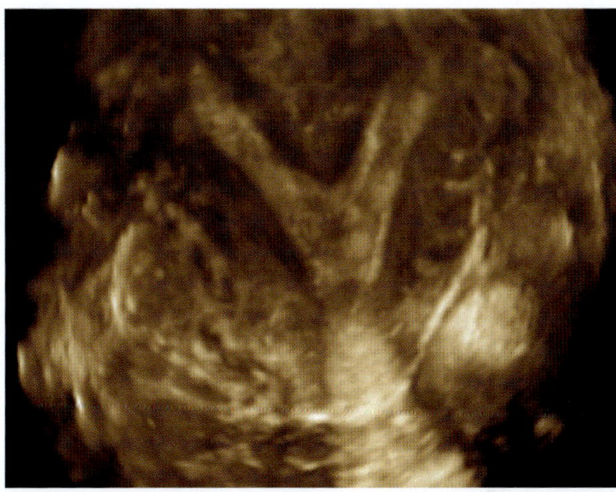

Fig. 2.8 Incomplete septate uterus: transvaginal 3D ultrasound showing endometrial echo as a "Y"-shaped image. The uterine cavity is separated in its upper half and shows a midline echo from its middle downward

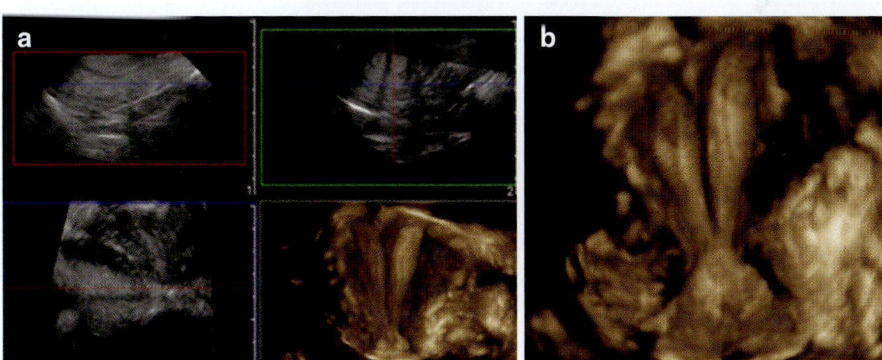

Fig. 2.9 Complete septate uterus: transvaginal 3D ultrasound showing endometrial echo as a "V"-shaped image; the uterine cavity with a hypoechoic middle septum. (**a**) 3D multiplanar images for 3D reconstruction 1,2,3. (**b**) Displaying a 3D image

Three-dimensional ultrasound scan can clearly show the septum in the uterine cavity of a septate uterus, its length, and its identification as a complete or incomplete septate uterus. Furthermore, it can also show the shape of the septum (Fig. 2.10a, b), its thickness at different levels of the uterus, etc. (Fig. 2.11a, b).

The clinical application of 3D ultrasonography gives a more accurate diagnosis of septate uterus and it is a direct visualization method. It also provides reliable information for the subsequent surgical treatment. The combination use of 3D ultrasound and saline hysterography (3D-HSG) further enhances the 3D ultrasound diagnosis. This will be easier to observe the morphology of the uterine septum and its relationship with the cervix and to determine the type of septate uterus. At the same time, it permits a timely diagnosis of any other associated uterine diseases such as endometrial polyps.

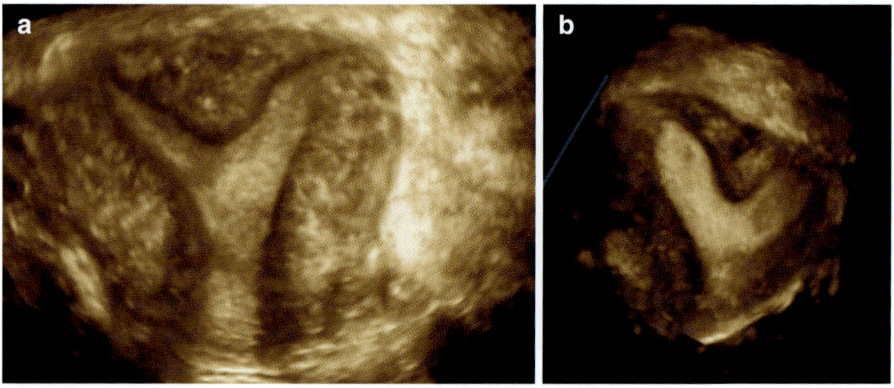

Fig. 2.10 3D transvaginal ultrasound of an incomplete septate uterus showing different shapes. (**a**) shows a wider septum. (**b**) shows a narrower and longer septum than the septum in (**a**)

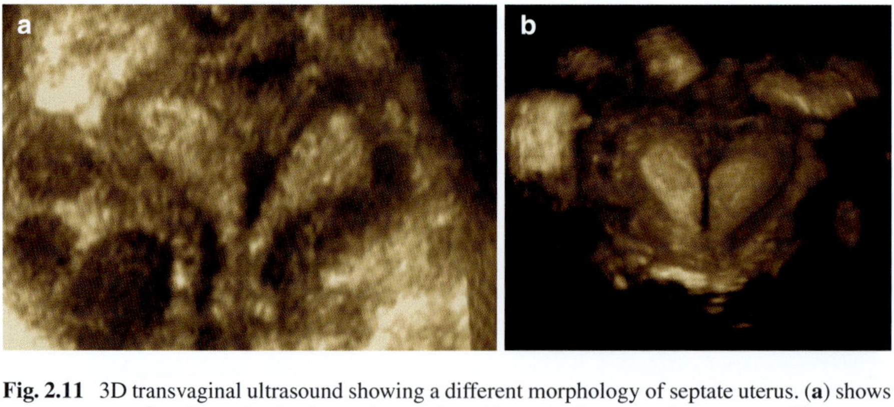

Fig. 2.11 3D transvaginal ultrasound showing a different morphology of septate uterus. (**a**) shows a septum extending from the fundus to the cervix with gradually narrowing septum. (**b**) shows a wider upper 1/3 septum and narrower lower 2/3 septum

Arcuate Uterus

It is a minor uterine anomaly in which the intervening septum at the uterine fundus is not fully absorbed after fusion. It has a localized muscular hypertrophy in the central part of the fundus and slightly protrudes into the uterine cavity from the fundus.

Ultrasound features: The cross section showed muscular thickening at the central part of the uterine fundus, slightly protruding into the uterine cavity. This feature is shown more clearly on the coronal plane in the 3D image (Fig. 2.12). The endometrium at the uterine fundus is shown as a curved concave, the angle between the two endometria > 90°; the shape and contour of the uterus are normal.

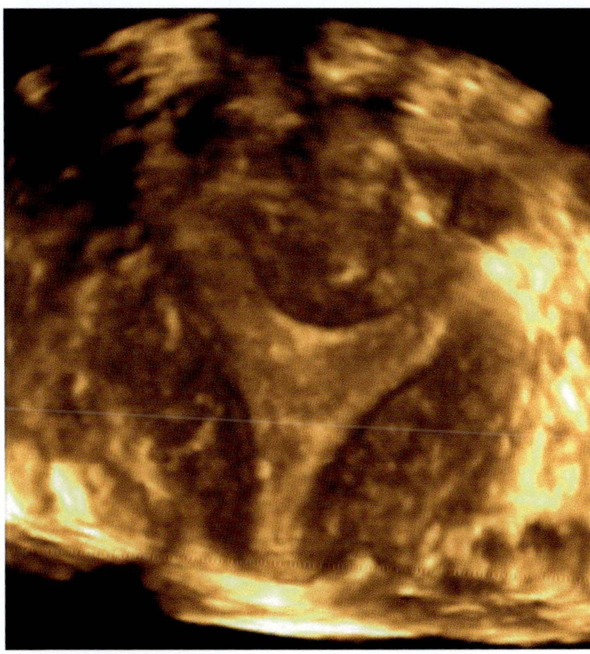

Fig. 2.12 Arcuate uterus: transvaginal 3D ultrasound image showing muscular thickening at the central part of the uterine fundus, slightly protruding into the uterine cavity, with a concave curved endometrium.

Other Ultrasound Features of Uterine Anomalies

1. Uterus didelphys may be misdiagnosed as uterine fibroids. Uterine fibroid sticks out from a uterus and may also change the shape of the uterus and be mistaken as a uterus didelphys. The key points for identification of uterine fibroid are the absence of endometrial echoes in uterine fibroid and the lower echo levels compared to the normal uterine myometrium.
2. Uterus didelphys is easier to diagnose, but the diagnosis of a septate uterus may be missed due to absence of changes in the uterine shape and contour. For this, a cross-sectional ultrasound observation may be particularly important to find whether there are two adjacent uterine endometrial echoes.
3. Identification of bicornuate uterus and uterus didelphys: The former has two complete uterine horns at an acute angle, and sometimes the bladder can show a "V"-shaped indentation, while the latter has two full uterine bodies, in between which may commonly show intestinal echoes.
4. Rudimentary horn may be misdiagnosed as a uterine fibroid or adnexal mass. The echo level should be carefully observed for presence of any uterine endometrial echoes. Rudimentary horn pregnancy is a dangerous problem which should attract great attention.
5. Transvaginal ultrasound probe has a higher frequency. As it is also closer to the uterus, it is of better value to observe bicornuate uterus, rudimentary horn, septate uterus, and a number of complex uterine anomalies; an abdominal ultrasound can show a complete uterine shape and contour, so its observation on the shape of a bicornuate uterus will be more comprehensive. Therefore, a combination of both ultrasound approaches can improve the diagnostic accuracy of detecting uterine anomalies, and avoid unnecessary false-negative diagnosis or misdiagnosed.

2.2.2 Ultrasound Features of Congenital Oblique Vaginal Septum Syndrome

Oblique vaginal septum syndrome is a congenital genital anomaly including uterus didelphys, double cervix, and a septum attaching to the vaginal wall extending obliquely from one side of the cervix; this often affects the patency of the ipsilateral cervix. An oblique vaginal septum is often associated with ipsilateral renal agenesis.

The clinical manifestations include painful menarche, lower abdominal pain or discomfort, excessive vaginal discharge with smell, or prolonged menstrual periods. In recent years, ultrasound examination has become the diagnostic method of choice, because of its advantages of being accurate, fast, real time, and noninvasive. Ultrasound examination shows not only the uterus and the cervix but also their number and shape and retention of blood in the vagina and the adnexa. It also gives an accurate diagnosis of renal agenesis.

Ultrasound Features

1. The uterus didelphys (with or without, particularly at the right side with retention of blood clots): The cross-sectional scan shows a fused cervix, with two separate uterine echoes which can be symmetrical or of different sizes; uterine endometrial echoes can be seen from both uterine cavities, with one of the uterine cavities often accompanied by retention of fluid (Fig. 2.13a–e).
2. A cystic mass on one side beneath one of the uterine bodies in fact is in the vagina. The cystic mass has clear edges, and within the cyst, there are sparsely to densely scattered dot-like echoes, above which are echoes from the connected cervix and the uterine body, as well as the contralateral cervix and its uterine body (Fig. 2.13a–d).
3. Abdominal ultrasound examination may reveal the absence of kidney on one side, mostly on the same side as the cystic mass (Fig. 2.13f). On the other side, the renal morphology was normal or with compensatory hypertrophy (Fig. 2.13g).
4. Perineal ultrasound examination can show the oblique vaginal septum, the distance between the oblique septum and the outer cervical opening, and even any hole in the oblique septum.

These ultrasound findings in patients with clinically dysmenorrhea and menstrual spotting can easily lead to a diagnosis of oblique vaginal septum syndrome.

2.2.2.1 The Differential Diagnoses of the Ultrasound Examination for Oblique Vaginal Septum

Oblique vaginal septum syndrome needs to be differentiated from imperforate hymen and ovarian cysts. ① Imperforate hymen may also manifest as cystic mass below the cervix, but the oblique vaginal septum syndrome mostly has uterus didelphys or septate uterus and can be associated with retention of fluid in one of the uterine cavities and renal agenesis on one side. Perineal ultrasound will help to diagnose the oblique vaginal septum. ② To differentiate it from an ovarian cyst, it is important to pay attention to the uterus. If there is a uterus didelphys anomaly, with a cystic mass below one of the uteri with sparse to dense dot-like echoes (hemorrhagic manifestation), together with renal agenesis on one side, it can easily differentiate it from an ovarian cyst.

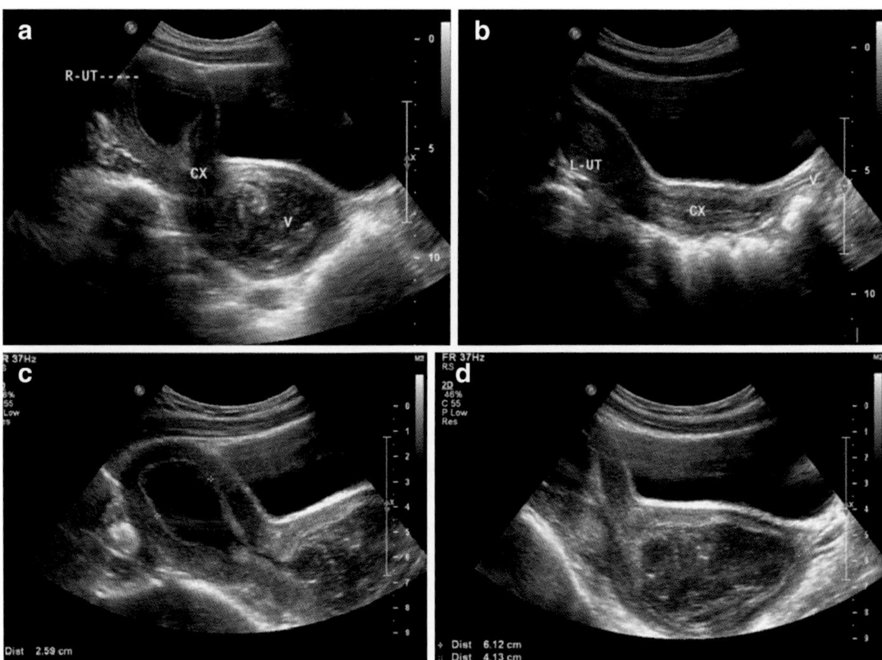

Fig. 2.13 Congenital oblique vaginal syndrome: a 12-year-old patient presenting with severe dysmenorrhea at menarche. Abdominal ultrasound scan shows a double uterus, double cervix, retention of blood in the right uterine cavity and vagina, as well as absence of the right kidney. (**a**) shows the right uterus and cervix; (**b**) shows the left uterus and cervix; (**c**) shows the right uterine cavity with echo-free zone of a thickness of 2.6 cm (due to retention of blood); (**d**) shows an echo-free zone in the vagina with a size of 6.2×4.1 cm, in which dense dots or strips echo can be seen; (**e**) shows the left uterine size (5.0×2.9 cm) with uterine endometrial echo; (**f**) shows an absence of the right kidney. (**g**) Compensatory hypertrophy of the left kidney

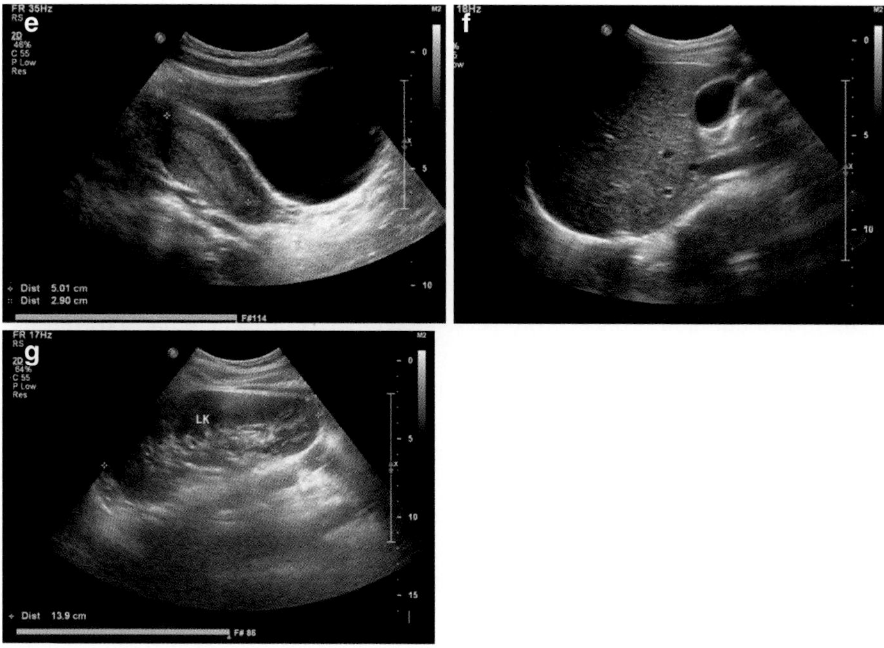

Fig. 2.13 (continued)

2.2.3 The Role of 3D Ultrasound in the Diagnosis of Uterine Anomalies

2D ultrasound, particularly transvaginal 2D ultrasound, can provide clear images of the uterus, the cervix, the adnexal region, and part of the vagina. Its value in the diagnosis of the female reproductive tract anomalies is unquestionable, but because 2D ultrasound cannot display the coronal sections of the uterus, to a certain extent, its ability to diagnose uterine anomaly can be limited. 3D ultrasound imaging is a good complement to the 2D ultrasound.

3D ultrasound can produce coronal section images of the uterus, showing the shape and contour of the entire uterus, uterine endometrial echo, and the shape of the uterine cavity. The high-resolution coronal imaging is easily reproducible and can display all the anatomical relationships from the uterine fundus, the uterine horns, and the cervix. It can provide accurate classification and differential diagnosis of the uterine anomalies. As reported in national and international literatures, 3D ultrasound diagnosis of uterine anomalies has a high diagnostic sensitivity and specificity of 92 and 100 %, respectively. Hence it can provide better information for the diagnosis and the plan for surgery. In particular for septate uterus, bicornuate uterus, and arcuate uterus, all of them are uterine anomalies that cannot be identified easily by 2D ultrasound. 3D ultrasound therefore has a higher ability for the diagnosis and differential diagnosis of reproductive tract anomalies. It is at present one of the best imaging methods for the diagnosis of uterine anomalies and is recommended for wider application.

2.2.4 Other Imaging Investigations

2.2.4.1 CT Examinations

CT scans have high spatial resolution and can therefore provide clear, constant anatomical images showing the cervix and the uterine body. In CT scanning, the normal uterus shows a higher density soft tissue images, which is of either circular, triangular, or spindle in shape, with a small low-density uterine cavity.

But CT scans can only provide cross-sectional imaging of the uterus, and the resolution on the soft tissue is low. It is therefore not ideal for showing the shapes of the uterus and has limited role in the diagnosis of some uterine anomalies; in addition, CT scans are not as simple as ultrasound examination; its higher ionizing radiation will be a hazard for women of childbearing age. For these reasons, CT scans are less often used for the diagnosis of uterine anomalies.

2.2.4.2 Magnetic Resonance Imaging (MRI)

Magnetic resonance imaging (MRI) has the advantages of high resolution on tissues, good contrast for soft tissues, more image parameters, non-ionizing radiation, etc. MRI can accurately distinguish between endometrial and myometrial signals and can have multi-directional scanning at any level for imaging. Its three-dimensional images can show the shape of the uterus and directly show the signals of septum and some other complications such as endometriosis, retrograde menstruation, and so on. As reported in the literatures, the sensitivity and specificity of MRI diagnosis of bicornuate uterus and septate uterus were 100 %. Therefore, MRI is the best imaging method in the diagnosis of uterine anomalies. It is the next important complementary method after 3D ultrasound examination. However, because of its high costs, it is rarely a routine application or the first-choice method.

MRI Manifestation of Uterine Anomalies

Rudimentary horn: It is a typical MRI image showing a banana-shaped body next to a developed uterus. The endometrial cavity of the uterus is reduced in size with reduced thickness. The best display image is at axial T2WI.

Uterus didelphys: A typical feature is double uterine cavities and double cervix. Each uterus has perfect anatomical signals.

Bicornuate uterus: A sagging uterine fundus with separated uterine horns. The best plane to show the contour at the uterine fundus is the coronal axial T1WI at the middle of the uterine body, while the best image to show the separate tissue signals is at axial T2WI.

Septate uterus: The center of the uterus shows some low-echo signals for the intervening fibrous tissue.

Arcuate uterus: At the central part of uterine fundus, there is thickened myometrium slightly protruding into the uterine cavity.

2.3 MRI Diagnosis of Female Genital Anomalies

Jingjing Lu

The incidence of female reproductive tract anomalies in the general population is about 7 %. For patients with recurrent miscarriages, it can reach up to 13–25 % [1]. Accurate preoperative diagnosis reaching a correct anatomical and morphological classification is important for the proper planning of surgery. It can effectively improve the management and avoid unnecessary invasive investigations. Appropriate imaging methods can directly and accurately demonstrate the reproductive tract anomalies. They have irreplaceable diagnostic value for the type of genital anomalies.

At present, the common imaging methods include hysterosalpingography (HSG), ultrasonography (US), and magnetic resonance imaging (MRI). HSG only shows the morphology of uterine cavity; the operation is relatively cumbersome and has low patient's compliance. Therefore its clinical application is very restricted. Ultrasonography is simple and low cost and has no radiation risk. It is the most popular imaging method currently used to diagnose female genital anomalies. However, it is highly operator dependent, and the image is not intuitive. In some anomalies such as rudimentary horn, the imaging display has great limitations.

With the increasing popularity of equipments and related technologies, magnetic resonance imaging has unique advantages in the female reproductive tract imaging. MRI has the advantages of high soft tissue resolution, multiplanar imaging, no radiation, and objective display of the reproductive tract anomalies. It has become the best imaging method for detecting genital anomalies. This chapter describes the clinical applications of MRI in the female genital anomalies.

2.3.1 The Recommended Imaging Criteria for MRI of the Female Reproductive System Anomalies

MRI uses the principle that different tissues possess relatively fixed and different relaxation times as T1 and T2, respectively, and they can be reflected in the MRI as the different intensities and signals in a black and white gray scale.

Before pelvic MRI scans, the general preparations include: The bladder must be at least half full to separate the uterus from the abdominal muscles, to push away the small intestines in the pelvic cavity so as to reduce peristaltic artifacts and optimize the image contrast. Before scanning, any metallic objects are to be removed from the body, including intrauterine devices. The lower abdomen should best be fixed by an abdominal belt to immobilize it. Whenever appropriate, a gel-like substance (such as the ultrasound coupling gel) should be instilled into patient's vagina. After the vagina is filled with gel, it will be much easier to get the image and observe the structures.

MRI examination of the female reproductive tract generally includes T1-weighted images (T1WI) and T2-weighted images (T2WI) collected from transverse, sagittal, and coronal planes. T2-weighted imaging is the main sequence of the female reproductive tract. T2-weighted images clearly demonstrate the shape of the uterus and its two adnexa and any other lesions when coupled with fat-suppression technology. Sagittal images show particularly ideal uterine diseases, and transverse and coronal images show more clearly the ovaries. T1-weighted images help to show the components of any lesion, such as bleeding, adipose tissue, and so on. T2W1 can distinguish the endometrium, junctional zone, and myometrium. These images can clearly show the different structures of uterine cavity, contour of the uterine fundus, various vaginal anomalies, and other pelvic lesions. Although T1W1 may not identify junctional zone in the uterus, but any retained blood within the uterine cavity and other pelvic complications which will be displayed by TIWI may provide useful diagnostic information.

The current recommendation of scanning sequence is shown in Table 2.1 [2, 3]. During the MRI scanning of female reproductive tract anomalies, the main MRI scanning position should be taken in accordance to the axis of the uterus, which is parallel to the long axis of the uterus and as well perpendicular to the long axis as short axis of the uterus. Sagittal views of the long axis of uterus, cervix, and vagina can show a better continuity display and allow an easy assessment of the ratio of the uterine body and cervix, as well as any obstructive vaginal anomaly. The T2WI images of the long axis of uterus are most valuable to make a diagnosis and classification of genital anomalies. The routine clinical application of sagittal T2W1 images shows obstructive vaginal anomalies. Large field-of-view coronal images have the advantages to show any associated kidney anomalies. About 29 % patients with Müllerian duct anomalies are associated with kidney anomalies, such as kidney agenesis, kidney hypoplasia, ectopic kidney, horseshoe kidney, and double renal pelvis or calyces [4]. Recently, the development of 3D T2-weighted sequences can capture thin slices T2 images, and after post-processing, it can display three-dimensional pictures of anomalies. This new 3D MRI techniques have been used by some medical institutions to replace the traditional two-dimensional MRI imaging [2].

In conclusion, MRI has high soft tissue resolution and multiplanar imaging capacity, and it produces no radiation. It is the best imaging method for reproductive tract anomalies after ultrasound imaging. Yet it is expensive, and it also has limitations to distinguish vaginal abnormalities from postoperative vaginal scar tissues.

Table 2.1 MRI sequences of female genital anomalies

Sequence	SSFSE	2D T2WI FRFSE (fat saturated)	2D T2WI FRFSE	3D T2WI FRFSE	TWI FSE (fat saturated)
Imaging plane	Coronal	Axial, sagittal	Oblique coronal	Axial	Axial
TR (ms)	1000–2000	2000–4000	2000–4000	2000–4000	600–700
TE (ms)	90	90	90	100	30
Echo train length	not applicable	16–20	16–20	126	4
Total imaging matrix	288×192	320×256	320×256	320×256×128	256×92
Field of FOV (cm)	40	26	26	26	26
Section thickness (mm)	6	5	5	1.4	5
Section space (mm)	0	1.5	1.5	0	1.5
Rationale	Give an overview display and detect the presence or absence of kidney		Be parallel to the long axis of the uterus to show the fundal contour	To obtain multiplanar reconstruction and curved planar reconstruction	To detect hemorrhage within the uterus or fallopian tube

2.3.2 *Classification of Female Genital Anomalies and Their MRI Features*

Müllerian ducts are the predecessors of the female genital system, which later develops into the uterus, cervix, and upper vagina. The embryo in its embryonic stage has a pair of longitudinal grooves in its posterior wall. This groove later transforms into a tube on each side as the Müllerian duct. Bilateral Müllerian ducts grow inward and downward and then fuse medially in the middle forming the uterus. If the proximal ends of the Müllerian ducts do not fuse properly or develop abnormally after fusion, these will result in female reproductive tract anomalies (or Müllerian duct anomalies).

2.3.2.1 Uterine Agenesis or Hypoplasia

Abnormal development of Müllerian ducts can lead to genital anomalies of the upper 2/3 of the vagina, the cervix, and the uterus, leading to their agenesis or hypoplasia. One type of this malformation is Mayer-Rokitansky-Kuster-Hauser syndrome (MRKH syndrome) (Fig. 2.14), which also represents the extreme form of Müllerian duct anomalies involving the proximal vagina, cervix, and uterus.

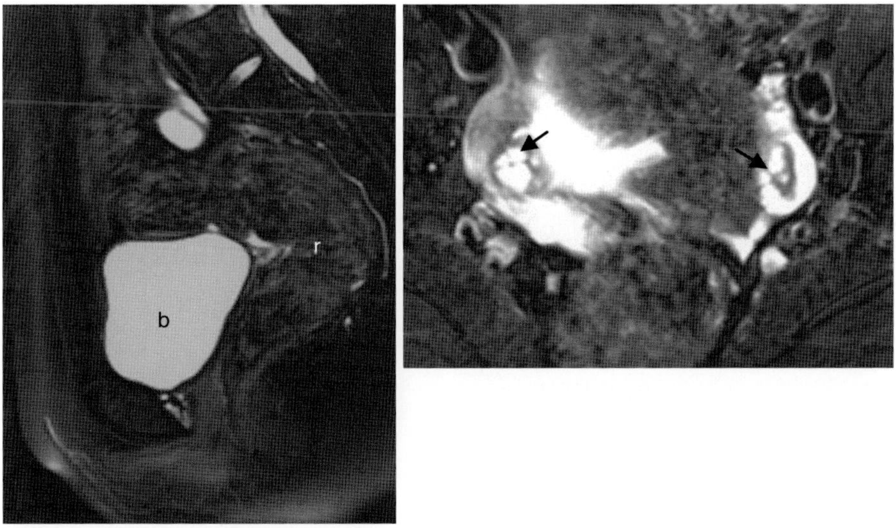

Fig. 2.14 Congenital absence of the uterus and vagina syndrome (Mayer-Rokitansky-Kuster-Hauser syndrome, MRKH syndrome). The *left* is fat-saturated sagittal T2-weighted image showed the complete absence of the cervix and uterus. Between the rectum (*r*) and bladder (*b*), normal vagina is invisible. The *right* is an axial T2-weighted image showing bilateral normal ovaries (*black arrows*)

For this type of genital anomalies, the sagittal T2-weighted images can be most intuitive and clear. Through the bladder and urethra in front and rectum behind, one can infer the location of the uterus, cervix, and vagina. In patients with complete agenesis of the uterus, the MRI images will show the absence of the uterus. A hypoplastic uterus will be displayed as a soft tissue mass in the pelvis, signal of which is consistent with a normal myometrium (the signal on T2-weighted images is slightly higher).

2.3.2.2 Unicornuate Uterus and Rudimentary Horn

Unicornuate uterus originates from one side of the Müllerian duct which is fully developed, while the other side is completely or nearly completely undeveloped. Approximately 40 % of these patients with unicornuate uterus have ipsilateral kidney anomaly. The most common anomaly is agenesis of the ipsilateral kidney (67 %) [4]. There are four subtypes of anomalies: (1) no contralateral rudimentary uterine horn, (2) rudimentary uterine horn with no endometrium or cavity, (3) rudimentary uterine horn with interconnected uterine cavities, and (4) rudimentary horn with no interconnected uterine cavities.

The MRI image of rudimentary horn will show a single "banana-like"-shaped horn on one side of the pelvis. The muscular wall signals and anatomy are normal. The ratio of endometrium to myometrium thickness is also normal. The clinical presentation of the rudimentary uterine horn varies with its subtype. If there is no endometrium, the entire rudimentary horn appears as diffuse low MRI signals. If endometrium exists in its cavity, the junctional zone of the rudimentary horn often presents well. If there is no communication between its endometrial cavity and the uterine cavity of the contralateral uterus, the rudimentary horn cavity will be gradually filled and distended with blood products after menarche (Fig. 2.15). The patient

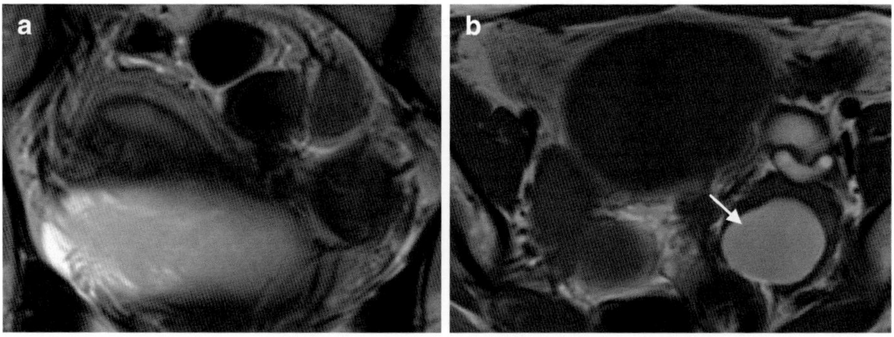

Fig. 2.15 (**a**) is a T2-weighted oblique coronary image and (**b**) is a T1-weighted axial image of the same person, in which a right unicornuate uterus and a left rudimentary uterus clearly appeared. The unicornuate uterus on the right is fully developed, and the distinct signal represents the three layers of the uterine body that can be easily detected; the rudimentary uterine on the left does not connect with the contralateral; hemorrhage within the cavity has a hyperintense signal upon T1 (*white arrow*)

will suffer from abdominal pain and pelvic endometriosis will develop in some patients because of retrograde blood flow into the peritoneal cavity. From the MRI images, it is important to distinguish the endometrial lining of the rudimentary horn, because the presence of functional intrauterine endometrium in this rudimentary horn is a high-risk factor for miscarriage, ectopic pregnancy, preterm delivery, and even uterine rupture [5].

2.3.2.3 Uterus Didelphys

Uterus didelphys arises when the uterine body and the cervical parts of both Müllerian ducts do not merge together. This results in double uterine bodies, double cervix, double vaginas, and/or single vagina. The MRI images will show two separate uterine bodies separated with a large angle toward both sides of the pelvis, associated with two cervices. The ratio of endometrium to myometrium and the junctional zone are normal. At the lower part of the uterus, there is an obvious cleft on the external contour (Fig. 2.16) probably suggestive of incomplete fusion (such as in a double uterus or bicornuate uterus), rather than from incomplete resorption after fusion (such as septate uterus). This is an important distinguishing feature of these two types of uterine anomalies.

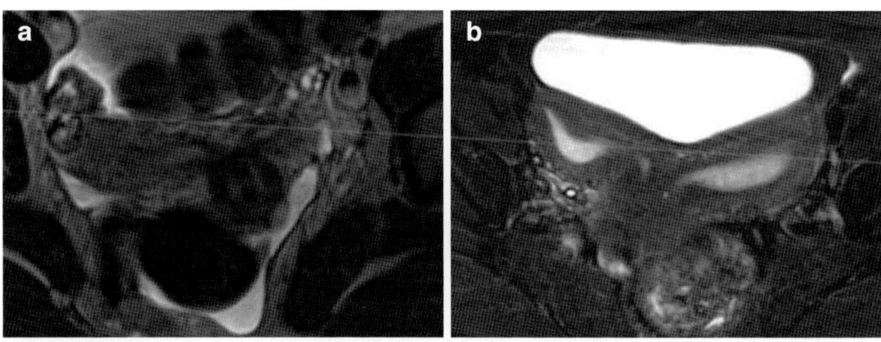

Fig. 2.16 (**a**) is an axial T2-weighted image showing a typical uterus didelphys, two widely splayed uterine horns with bilateral, non-fused, fully developed cervices, which is critical for distinction from bicornuate uterus. (**b**) is a uterus didelphys which has two relatively separate cavities

Three-quarters of these patients have repetition of the proximal end of the vagina. If there is an oblique vaginal septum on one side, it can cause blood-filled uterine cavity on the same side of the septum. Blood products often show high MRI signal on T1-weighted images. Congenital oblique vaginal septum syndrome (i.e., the Herlyn-Werner-Wunderlich syndrome, HWW syndrome) is a rare congenital disorder of the genitourinary system, involving the Müllerian and Wolffian ducts. The clinical triad includes (1) double uterus, (2) vagina hemi-obstruction, and (3) ipsilateral renal agenesis (Fig. 2.17). MRI is a noninvasive imaging method which is very sensitive to demonstrate this syndrome as well as show its anatomical anomalies and concurrent pathological changes [6].

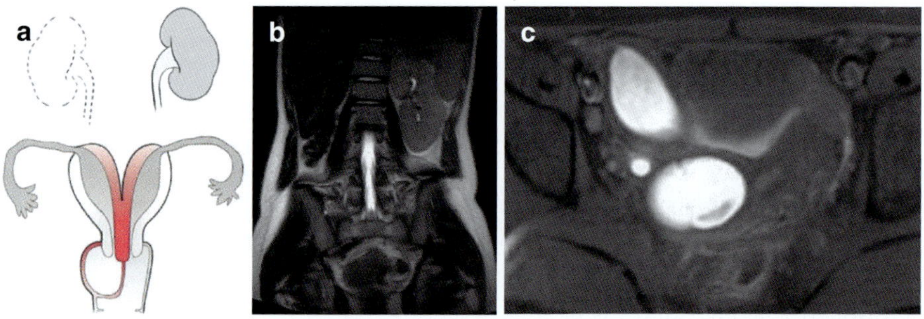

Fig. 2.17 Schematic oblique vaginal septum syndrome and MRI images. (**a**) A schematic view showing a double uterus with unilateral renal agenesis. As the cavity of the uterus and cavity of oblique vaginal septum communicate through the cervix, outflow obstruction of the uterine cavity due to the oblique septum will cause blood retention behind the septum and the uterine cavity. The contralateral uterus, cervix, and kidney appear normal. (**b**) An axial T1-weighted MRI image showing hemorrhage is visible in the right uterine cavity and in the vagina above the oblique vaginal septum. (**c**) A coronal T2-weighted image showing the right kidney is absent

2.3.2.4 Bicornuate Uterus

Bicornuate uterus is also due to incomplete fusion of the bilateral Müllerian ducts. It accounts for 10 % of all Müllerian duct anomalies. The MRI image of bicornuate uterus also shows a characteristic cleft over the external contour at the lower part of the uterus.

Normal double horns can be seen on the MRI image combined with normal anatomical structure (Fig. 2.18). Whether the mid-lower horn or uterine body is fused or not is the pinpoint in differentiation between uterus didelphys and bicornuate uterus. Between two symmetrical intrauterine cavities, there is a visible soft tissue separating the horns, which is also the difference between bicornuate uterus and a double uterus. While it's relatively difficult to accurately distinguish a bicornuate bicollis uterus from a uterus didelphys upon MRI, fortunately, the treatment strategy is not too much different between this two anomalies, in view of a surgical intervention that is not usually indicated for patients with fusion anomalies, but with reabsorption anomalies like septate uterus.

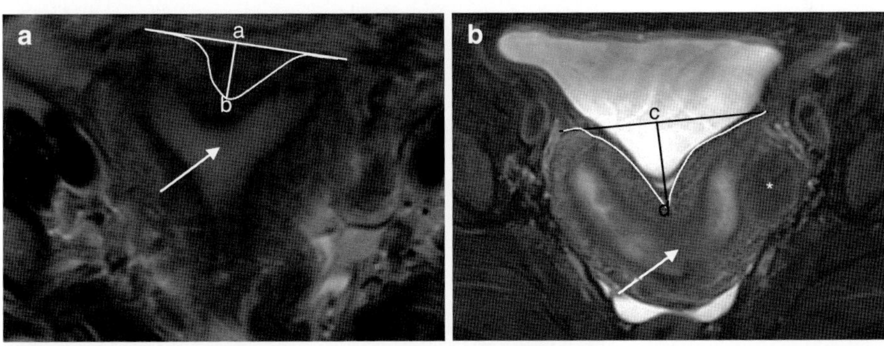

Fig. 2.18 (**a**, **b**) are two cases of bicornuate uterus, characterized by the presence of a fundal clef more than 1 cm (indicated by the *white line ab* and *black line cd*). The outer contour of the uterine is roughly outlined by the *curved line*. Two separate uterine horns with fusion of the mid-lower uterine body (*white arrow*) are distinctly manifested. The accompanying round-like leiomyoma (*) upon the left horn in (**b**) can be easily identified

2.3.2.5 Septate Uterus

Septate uterus is the most common, accounting for 55 % of the duct anomalies [7]. It is important to distinguish between it and the bicornuate uterus. A midline longitudinal septum arises from the fundus of the uterus, which is due to incomplete resorption of the fused septum in the uterus.

On MRI image, the uterus is of normal size. The external contour of the fundus of the uterus is similar to that of a normal uterus (Fig. 2.19); this is the most important point to distinguish a septate uterus from a bicornuate uterus. The features in ultrasound examination can be used as a standard reference (Fig. 2.20). The longitudinal septum may be incomplete or complete septum. A complete longitudinal uterine septum extends from the fundus to the external os of the cervix. In 25 % of patients, it can extend to the vagina. Uterine septum can have different lengths and tissue components, with various proportions of fibrous tissues and muscle tissues.

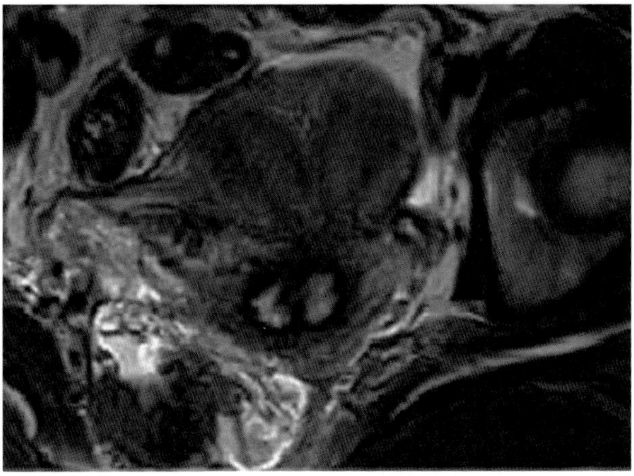

Fig. 2.19 A complete septate uterus: the external contour of the fundus is normal. The septum extends from the uterine fundus to the external cervical os

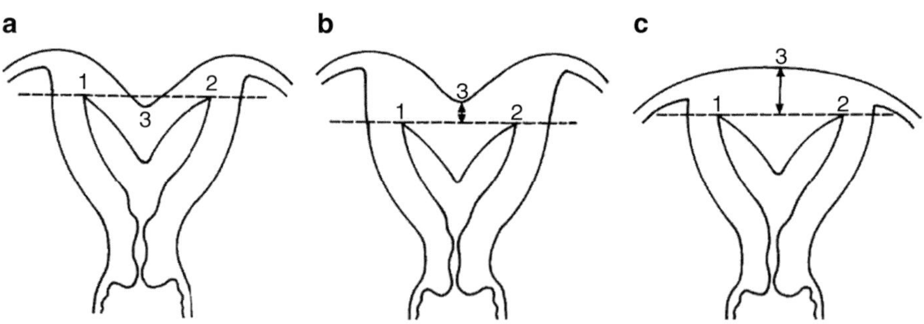

Fig. 2.20 Classification criteria for US differentiation of septate from bicornuate uteri. (**a**) When apex (*3*) of the fundal external contour occurs below a straight line between the tubal ostia (*1*, *2*) or (**b**) 5 mm (*arrow*) above it, the uterus is bicornuate. (**c**) When apex is more than 5 mm (*arrow*) above the line, uterus is septate

2.3.2.6 Arcuate Uterus

Arcuate uterus occurs when the septa of the uterus and vagina have almost completely absorbed. In the MRI image, the fundus of the uterus shows slightly convex internal contour toward the uterine cavity. Arcuate uterus is a mild Müllerian duct anomaly. It usually does not cause problems in pregnancy.

On a MRI image, the uterine size is normal. The uterus has a wider uterine cavity, with a saddle-shaped bulge (Fig. 2.21), protruding into the endometrial cavity. The MRI signals of the protruding tissue are similar to the uterine myometrium. The contour of the fundus is also normal.

The above anomalies are classified according to the genital anomaly classification of the American Fertility Society's definition in 1988. The typical MRI anomalies are briefly described. However, there are limitations of this classification, because there are no definition and classification of vaginal anomalies. Some complex anomalies have also been defined across different anomaly groups with the classification. As such, we cannot have an absolute pathological changes defined into any classification. It is then acceptable to have a clear and comprehensive description of the anomalies. MRI imaging for female reproductive tract anomalies is intuitive and reliable. Following our advancing MRI technology and our increased awareness of anomalies, MRI will play an increasingly important role in the diagnosis, preoperative planning, and postoperative follow-up of the female reproductive system anomalies.

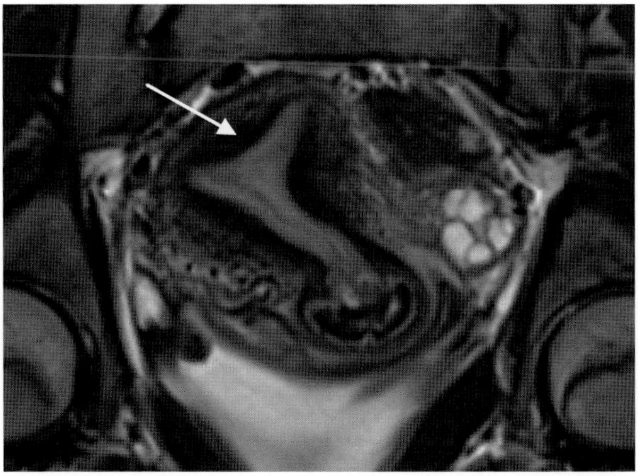

Fig. 2.21 The T2-weighted image of an arcuate uterus with a slightly convexed fundus. The broad-based myometrium bulge toward the endometrial cavity (*white arrow*)

References

1. Chan YY, et al. The prevalence of congenital uterine anomalies in unselected and high-risk populations: a systematic review. Hum Reprod Update. 2011;17(6):761–71.
2. Behr SC, Courtier JL, Qayyum A. Imaging of Mullerian duct anomalies. Radiographics. 2012;32(6):E233–50.
3. Robbins JB, et al. MRI of pregnancy-related issues: Mullerian duct anomalies. AJR Am J Roentgenol. 2012;198(2):302–10.
4. Li S, et al. Association of renal agenesis and Mullerian duct anomalies. J Comput Assist Tomogr. 2000;24(6):829–34.
5. Jayasinghe Y, et al. The presentation and early diagnosis of the rudimentary uterine horn. Obstet Gynecol. 2005;105(6):1456–67.
6. Sen KK, Balasubramaniam D, Kanagaraj V. Magnetic resonance imaging in obstructive Mullerian anomalies. J Hum Reprod Sci. 2013;6(2):162–4.
7. Homer HA, Li TC, Cooke ID. The septate uterus: a review of management and reproductive outcome. Fertil Steril. 2000;73(1):1–14.

Suggested Reading

Dykes TM, Siegel C, Dodson W. Imaging of congenital uterine anomalies: review and self-assessment module. AJR Am J Roentgenol. 2007;189:S1–10.

Grimbizis GF, Gordts S, Di Spiezio Sardo A, et al. The ESHRE/ESGE consensus on the classification of female genital tract congenital anomalies. Hum Reprod. 2013;28(8):2032–44.

Jinghe Lang. Adolescent gynecology. Beijing: People's Military Medical Press; 2011. p. 19–44.

Qinsheng Ge. Practical female reproductive endocrinology. Beijing: Scientific and Technological Literature Publishing House; 2001. p. 275–319.

Troiano RN, McCarthy SM. Müllerian duct anomalies: imaging and clinical issues1. Radiology. 2004;233:19–34.

Chapter 3
Abnormal Development of External Genitalia

Fang Jiang, Qinjie Tian, Shu Wang, and Lan Zhu

3.1 Abnormal Hymen

Fang Jiang and Lan Zhu

The hymen is a layer of mucosal membrane located at the vaginal opening, with squamous epithelium covering its outer and inner surfaces. In between these surfaces, it contains connective tissue, blood vessels, and nerve endings. During its development, abnormal cavity formation at the urogenital sinus will lead to various anomalies which include imperforate hymen, microperforate hymen, septate hymen, and cribriform hymen (Fig. 3.1)

F. Jiang • Q. Tian • S. Wang • L. Zhu (✉)
Department of Obstetrics and Gynecology, Peking Union Medical College Hospital,
No. 1 Shuaifuyuan, Beijing 100730, P. R. China
e-mail: zhu_julie@sina.com; qinjietn@sohu.com

© Springer Science+Business Media Dordrecht 2015
L. Zhu et al. (eds.), *Atlas of Surgical Correction of Female Genital Malformation*,
DOI 10.1007/978-94-017-7246-4_3

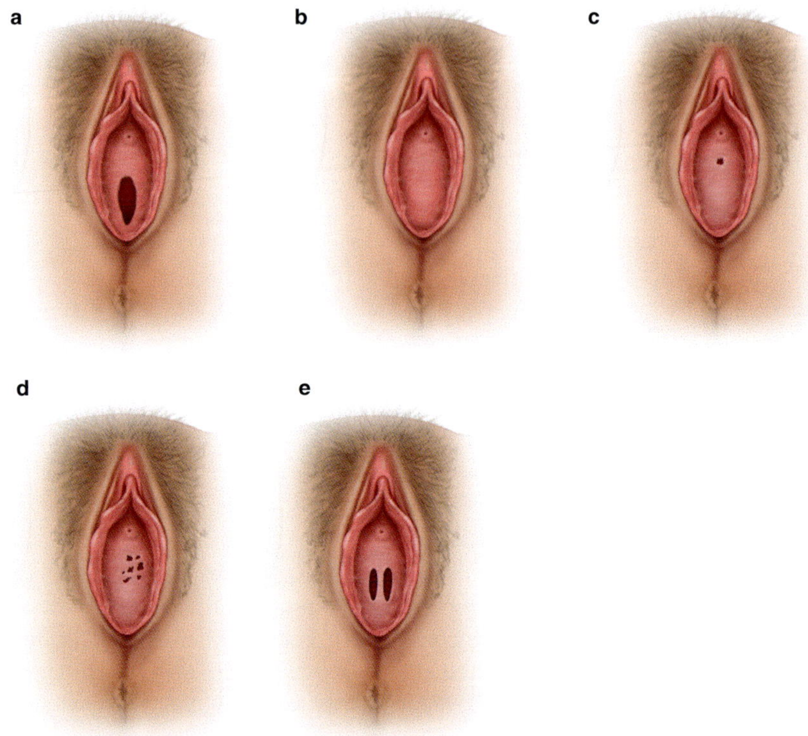

Fig. 3.1 Congenital anomalies of the hymen. (**a**) Normal hymen; (**b**) incomplete perforated hymen; (**c**) microperforate hymen; (**d**) cribriform hymen; (**e**) septate hymen

3.1.1 Diagnostic Criteria

3.1.1.1 Imperforate Hymen

Imperforate hymen is also known as nonporous hymen. The incidence of imperforate hymen is about 0.015 %. Imperforate hymen mainly obstructs the discharge of vaginal secretions. It may be asymptomatic at childhood due to minimal vaginal secretions, but at puberty, as both the vaginal and cervical secretions gradually increase, they accumulate in the vagina and lead to a sense of heaviness in the lower abdomen. After menarche, as the menstrual blood cannot drain out, it accumulates in the vagina forming a vaginal hematoma after several menstruations. Subsequently, it may lead to uterine and tubal hematomas, and eventually retrograde flow will enter into the pelvic cavity forming pelvic hematomas. Clinical symptoms are obvious with a cyclical lower abdominal pain, which progressively increases in intensity.

On gynecological examination, a bulging hymen can be seen, with a purple blue surface; on rectal examination, a vaginal mass bulging into the rectum is felt as a palpable pelvic mass. With a finger pressing on the vaginal mass, the bulging hymen can be made more obvious. Ultrasound scan may show accumulated fluid in the vagina and even in the uterine cavity.

3.1.1.2 Microperforate Hymen

It is a rare anomaly. There is a film covering the vaginal opening with just a pin hole opening as first described by Capraro in 1968 [1]. Since the pin hole is often difficult to detect, it is often misdiagnosed as an imperforate hymen. According to the sizes of the pin hole, the presenting symptoms will be different. Some patients have periodic menstruations with moderate amount of menstrual blood outflow, but a lot of blood still accumulates in the vagina; sometimes the periods are irregular; some patients presented with delayed menarche, with their chief complaints that include periodic abdominal pain and painful pelvic mass due to hematoma formation [2]. Microperforate or imperforate hymen can occur as an isolated anomaly, but it can also be associated with other reproductive tract anomalies, such as bicornuate uterus, vestibular anomalies, and anal atresia [3].

Similar to imperforate hymen, microperforate hymen can cause reflux of vaginal secretions and blood into the peritoneal cavity forming a pelvic mass. Unlike imperforate hymen, it will also cause recurrent urinary tract infections and sometimes a pelvic abscess. It is because the pinhole opening can have communication to the outside, through which bacteria will enter and multiply in the accumulated effusion or blood in the vagina or the pelvis leading a pelvic abscess. Bacteria can also migrate out of the vaginal opening, enter into the urethra, and cause recurrent urinary tract infections. On the contrary, patients with imperforate hymen do not have these presentations because their vaginas do not communicate with the outside [4]. The microperforate hymen is mainly diagnosed by examination under general anesthesia, and nowadays, fiber-optic hysteroscopy can be useful in its diagnosis together with simultaneous examination of any anomalies in the vagina and cervix [5].

3.1.2 Indication and Timing of Surgery

Surgery may be performed at any age. The ideal times are at the postneonatal period, puberty, or before menarche. As the development of hematocolpos can cause blood accumulation in the vagina, uterus, and fallopian tubes, followed by secondary endometriosis or pelvic infection, therefore, once hymen anomalies is diagnosed, surgery should be performed as soon as possible.

3.1.3 Surgical Contraindications

Vaginal atresia or the congenital absence of a vagina and other congenital anomalies should be ruled out before performing the surgery to incise the hymen. Surgery must be after a proper diagnosis of other anomalies (Fig. 3.2).

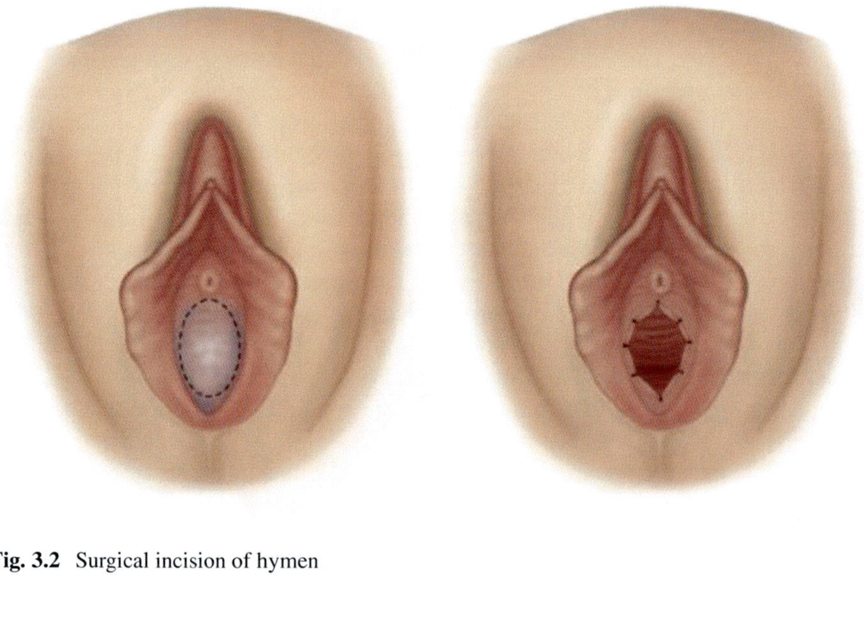

Fig. 3.2 Surgical incision of hymen

3.1.4 *Preparative Preparation*

Preoperative preparation is similar to other vulval surgery with routine cleansing and antiseptic preparation of the vulva.

3.1.5 *Anesthesia and Positioning*

The patient is placed in a lithotomy position. Local infiltration with anesthetic or intravenous anesthesia or general anesthesia can be used.

3.1.6 *Surgical Procedure*

Many literatures recommend the same surgical treatment for both microperforate and imperforate hymen. This includes surgical incision and removal of the accumulated blood in the vagina. After the surgery, patients will have significantly improved pregnancy rate and quality of life.

3.1.6.1 Incision

A metal urinary catheter should be used if possible to guide its position to avoid bladder injury. The surgeon should wear double gloves and insert the index finger of the left hand into the anus pressing towards the vagina for guidance, so as to avoid injury to the rectum. The incision should be at the most prominent part of the bulging hymen, though it will depend on the personal choice. The incision can be a "cross" incision, a vertical incision or a puncture incision at the center. Some surgeons think that it should begin with a small incision (especially for a thickened hymen), so as to reduce the rate of blood flow and hence to prevent vasovagal reaction due to the sudden decompression of the vaginal hematoma. Then, the outer glove of the left hand is removed to examine if the vaginal opening can accommodate one finger. Attention should be paid to avoid damaging the urethra and rectum during surgery. Finally, the vagina and cervix should be examined for other associated anomalies.

3.1.6.2 Evacuation of Hematoma

After opening the imperforate hymen, the retained menstrual blood will drain off. Any blood should be mopped up with gauze, and the cervix can now be visualized and examined. In the presence of a cervical adhesion or stenosis, a small uterine dilator is used to discharge any intrauterine blood retention. Tubal blood collection will gradually drain out following the operation. The abdomen should not be pressed or kneaded to avoid rupture of a hematoma or to force more retained blood flowing into the peritoneal cavity.

3.1.6.3 Suturing Edges of the Incisions

Any redundant hymen tissue should be cut off from the incision wounds. Absorbable sutures are used to suture the edges, while a very thin hymen wound without bleeding may not require suturing. In the literatures, absorbable sutures No. 3 "0" or No. 4 "0" are recommended to suture the wound edges or to cauterize wound edges with diathermy, so as to avoid wound adhesion with subsequent stenosis.

3.1.7 Postoperative Management

1. Rest in a semisupine position is recommended, but patient is encouraged to sit up or to get out of bed to facilitate the drainage of any residual retained blood.
2. It is important to maintain good vulval hygiene. Sitz bath or vaginal lavage is necessary for one week to avoid ascending infection. Prophylactic antibiotic is not often used.
3. Patient can be discharged home on postoperative day 2 if she is fit for discharge.
4. After 6–8 weeks, the uterus and the fallopian tubes will recover completely to their normal conditions. Any persistent enlargement of the fallopian tubes or persistent symptoms of peritoneal irritation should require further investigations.

3.2 Virilization of the External Genitalia

Qinjie Tian

3.2.1 Perineal Incision and Repair

3.2.1.1 Diagnostic Criteria

Female patients with a normal vagina but with a high perineal body or fused labia minora would have their vaginal opening completely or partially obliterated, resulting in poor menstrual blood flow or poor sex life. This vulval anomaly is mainly due to abnormal androgenic influence. Clinically it can be manifested as ambiguous external genitalia, labial fusion, and common vaginal and urethral opening. Prader classified external genital anomalies into the five types according to the varying degrees of virilization of the external genitalia: As illustrated by the following photos (Fig. 3.3), these types are described as:

Type I: Larger clitoris, with normal vagina and urethral openings.

Type II: Larger clitoris, with a funnel-shaped vaginal opening, but the openings for the vagina and urethra are still separated.

Type III: Significantly enlarged clitoris, both the vagina and urethra open from a common urogenital sinus.

Type IV: Significantly enlarged clitoris like a penis, the base of the penis is at the urogenital sinus, similar to hypospadias with fusion of the reproductive uplifted part.

Type V: Clitoris looks like a penis with the urethral opening at the penis tip. There is a complete fusion of the reproductive uplifted part; it is often mistaken as a male penis with cryptorchidism and hypospadias.

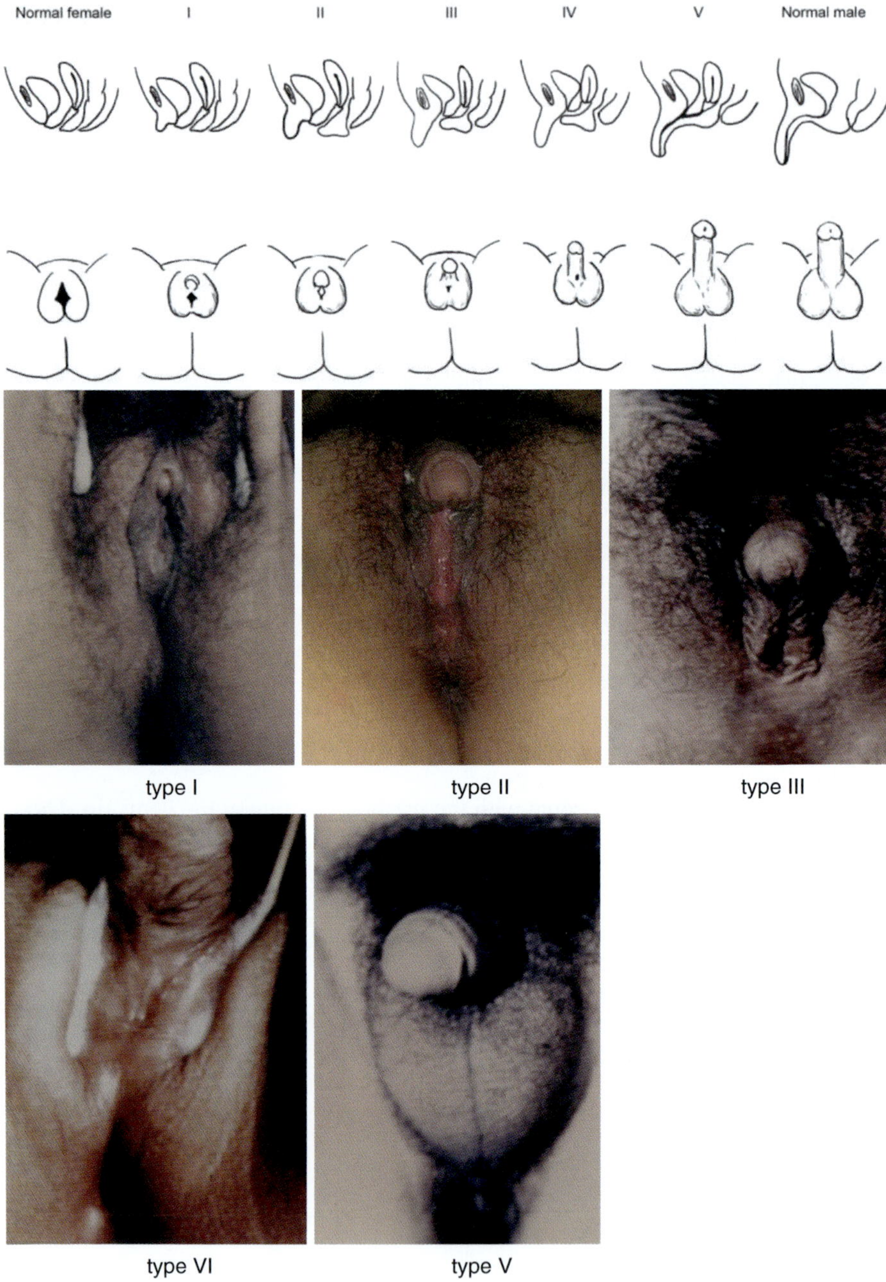

Fig. 3.3 Appearances of the external genitalia of normal female, 5 types of various degrees of virilisation and normal male

3.2.1.2 Operative Indications

Diagnosis can be easily made and accurately confirmed by examination. They are patients with a normal vagina and high vulval body or fusion of labia minora.

3.2.1.3 Timing of Surgery

1. After menarche, patient presented with poor menstrual flow.
2. Patient with difficult or impossible sexual intercourse.
3. Patient for clitoral surgery.

3.2.1.4 Preoperative Preparation

Routine vulval skin cleaning and antiseptic preparation are performed.

3.2.1.5 Anesthesia

Local anesthesia is used for the labial incision and repair. If there is also a simultaneous corrective surgery for the clitoris or for vaginoplasty, general anesthesia or epidural anesthesia is recommended for these procedures.

3.2.1.6 Position

Patient is placed in a lithotomy position same as other vaginal surgery.

3.2.2 Surgical Procedures

1. The vulva is disinfected and the bladder is catheterized.
2. The perineal body is identified, and a midline incision is performed down to the lower vaginal opening.
3. The vertical incision exposes the vaginal opening. The cut wound is sutured horizontally with 3/0 or 4/0 absorbable interrupted sutures (Fig. 3.4).

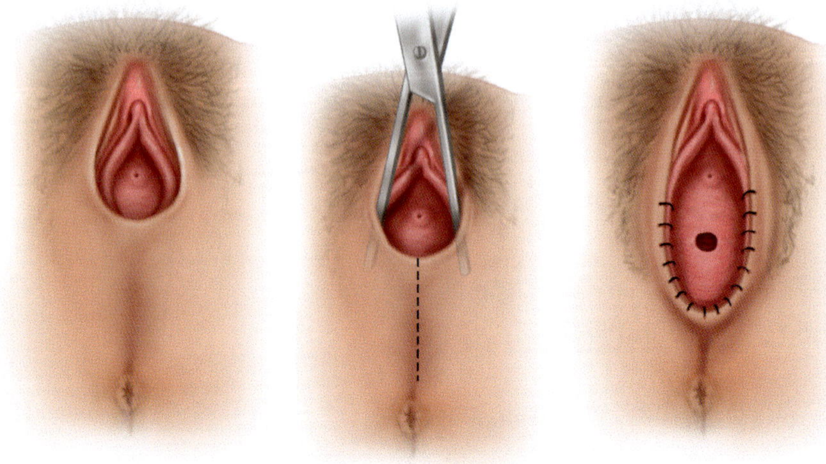

Fig. 3.4 Perineal incision and repair of abnormal external genitalia with common vaginal and urethral opening as described in Sect. 3.2.2

3.2.2.1 Postoperative Management

1. The vulva should be kept clean to prevent infection.
2. The labial wounds should be separated and prevented from adhesion formation.

3.2.2.2 Key Points of Surgical Techniques

1. Prevention of urethral injury is important.
2. After this vulval operation, the labia should be prevented from re-adhesion.

3.2.3 Surgical Excision of Long Clitoris and Repair

The clitoris is located between the top ends of the labia minora, and at the meeting point of the upper ends of the labia majora. It is a small cylindrical organ about 1.5–3.5 cm long, surrounded by foreskin. The swollen tip is called the glans clitoris. Under the skin, there is a bunch of erectile tissue. The erectile tissue is composed of cavernous tissue (there are two erectile clitoris cavernosa, similar to a male penis, and it is divided into head, body, and feet), with rich venous plexus and nerve endings. Therefore, it is very sensitive and bleeds easily after injury.

The size of the clitoris head is about 3–4 mm wide and 4–5 mm long, smaller than the eraser head of a pencil. There may be ethnic differences. The clitoris is a sensitive organ which plays an important role in achieving and maintaining sexual satisfaction and orgasm. The simple clitoral excision in the past has been abandoned and changed to clitoral plastic surgery which would keep the blood vessels and nerves.

3.2.3.1 Diagnostic Criteria

The cause of an enlarged clitoris must be accurately diagnosed before surgery. In many women, the common causes for an enlarged clitoris include:

1. Excessive androgen: For patients of female sex genotype (46, XX), the most common cause is congenital adrenal hyperplasia, followed by excessive exogenous androgen exposure during early pregnancy.
2. Lack of androgen: For patients of male sex genotype (46, XY), it is due to incomplete androgen insensitivity syndrome, and in some rare cases, it is the testicular regression or partial 17α-hydroxylase deficiency.
3. Failure of gonadal differentiation: True hermaphroditism (for chromosome 46, XX or 46, XY) and 45, X/46, XY gonadal dysgenesis are common.

3.2.3.2 Surgical Indication

1. Any female patient, who is confirmed to have genital anomalies with a large clitoris.
2. She is willing and requesting to live as a woman.

3.2.3.3 Timing of Surgery

1. After an accurate diagnosis, the surgical timing will depend on the woman's sex life and her cause of anomalies.
2. After treatment, androgen level should be monitored and controlled within that of a normal woman, or at the time of genital plastic surgery, surgical removal of male gonads should be performed.

3.2.3.4 Preoperative Preparation

The cleaning and antiseptic preparation of the vulva before operation is performed to avoid infection.

3.2.3.5 Anesthesia

Patient will require either general anesthesia or epidural anesthesia.

3.2.3.6 Position

Patient should be positioned in a lithotomy position as in other vaginal surgery.

3.2.3.7 Surgical Procedures

1. Patient is positioned in a lithotomy position, followed by routine vulval disinfection, sterile strapping, and bladder catheterization.
2. A stitch is anchored at the anterior midline position of the foreskin of the clitoris to serve as a marker stitch.
3. The dorsum of the foreskin is marked with a line pen for wound incision about 0.5 cm along the root of foreskin if the labia minora appear normal and satisfactory. If plastic surgery for the labia minora is necessary, a straight line is drawn from the front edge of the foreskin to the root of the clitoris.
4. Diluted norepinephrine 4 mg in 100 ml normal saline is injected subcutaneously to reduce bleeding.
5. The epidermis and dermis along the marked line are incised; the subcutaneous fat tissue is cut to expose the clitoral corpus cavernosum. Use a small Kelly

clamp, to dissect bluntly laterally from the midline over the cavernosum and to separate, free, and avoid any injury to the vessels and nerve fibers on the dorsal surface of the clitoris, until the dissection reaching the pubis symphysis.

6. The cavernosum body at the pubic symphysis is cut at where they fork out, ligated, and sutured to stop bleeding.
7. The cavernosum head is also freed, separated, and ligated. It is important to avoid injury of the blood and nerve plexus on the dorsal surface of the clitoris.
8. The cavernous ends at the pubic symphysis is inspected carefully, and any bleeding stopped meticulously. The cavernous stumps are placed and fixed to the fascia over the pubic symphysis, and both opposite ends are approximated.
9. If the glans still appears large, a symmetrical triangular tissue can be removed at the bottom part to reduce the size of the glans. If necessary, remove more clitoral tissue to further reduce the size.
10. The midpoint edge of the clitoris is used as a guide; the skin around the clitoris is sutured with 3/0 or 4/0 absorbable interrupted sutures. The foreskin can be used to form a part of the labia minora. If there are plenty of dead spaces around the clitoris, a small drainage may be necessary (Fig. 3.5).

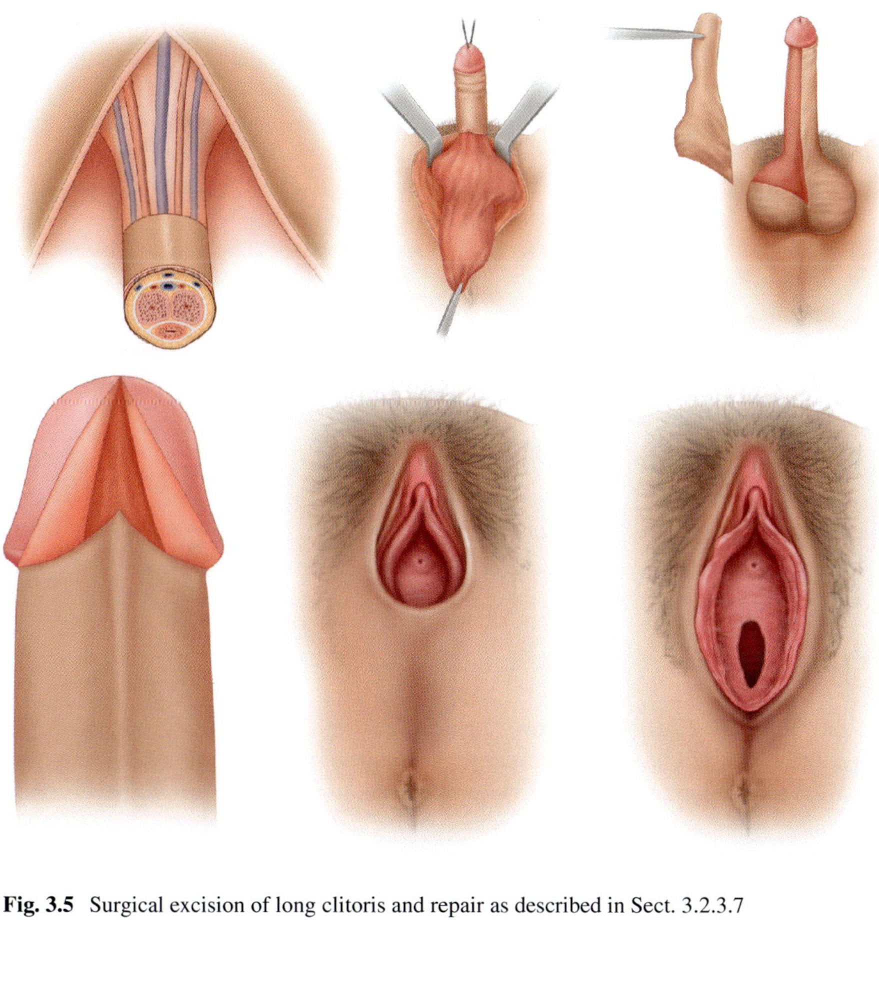

Fig. 3.5 Surgical excision of long clitoris and repair as described in Sect. 3.2.3.7

3.2.3.8 Postoperative Management

1. The urinary catheter is kept in situ for 2–3 days to avoid retention of urine due to pain and hence fear to urinate.
2. Local wound pain should be treated symptomatically.
3. Any blood oozing from the wound should be treated by applying topical hemostatic agents or local pressure.
4. Patient should be allowed to get out of bed on the second day after surgery, to wash the perineum twice a day and also after bowel opens.
5. Broad-spectrum antibiotics are used to prevent infection after surgery.
6. Sexual intercourse is prohibited for 1 month after surgery.

3.2.3.9 Key Points of Surgical Techniques

1. The clitoris is the most important sexually sensitive organ especially the glans clitoris which is full of nerve endings. Woman's clitoris is equivalent to a man's penis, and the clitoral glans is equivalent to the glans penis. Therefore, care must be taken to preserve its blood vessels and nerves.
2. Preoperative surgical procedures should be well planned ahead, as to have the idea on how to form the new labia minora and to reduce clitoral glans to a desirable size.
3. During the operation, the damage to the vascular and nerve plexuses of the clitoris should be avoided as far as possible. Starting from the anterior midline of the clitoris, the vascular and nerve plexuses at the subcutaneous skin are freed and lifted away from the cavernous body, to avoid their injuries.
4. The lateral side of clitoral corpus cavernosum has small subcutaneous blood vessels. Therefore, hemostasis should be strictly controlled to prevent postoperative hematoma. There are deep arteries within the cavernosum, which after excision should be tightly ligated to prevent bleeding.

3.3 Labial Fusion/Adhesion

Shu Wang and Lan Zhu

3.3.1 Diagnosis

3.3.1.1 Symptoms

Patients with labial fusion will have normal menstruation at puberty, but menstrual blood and urine will be noticed coming out from the same opening which might be mistaken as "cyclical hematuria"; patients also complain of failure to have sexual intercourse as the penis cannot penetrate into the vagina.

In addition, due to different extents of fusion of the labia minora, the degree of covering to the vaginal opening can be different. If it is a narrow opening close to the pubic symphysis, the outflow of urine and blood is likely to be sluggish. Sometimes even before puberty, pelvic mass will form as a result of urine reflux to the vagina or uterus cavity. Worse still, the obstruction by the distended vagina and uterus can lead to hydroureters and hydronephrosis. After menarche, it may be associated with retention of blood in the vagina or uterine cavity [6–8] leading to obstruction of the lower urinary tract and recurrent urinary tract infections.

3.3.1.2 Examination

At the perineum, there are two small openings. An anterior hole-like opening is located at the normal urethral opening position; the posterior opening is the anal opening. They are in their normal positions. With a metal urinary probe, the anterior opening can be probed into and lead to some urine outflow, thus confirming it as the urethral opening. The metal probe can then be withdrawn just behind the anterior small opening and move downwards in a perpendicular direction towards the anus; it can be felt probing into the vagina. Between the anterior urethral and anal openings, there is a layer of normal perineal skin covering the hidden vaginal opening. Gynecological examination can reveal a normal uterus, normal cervix, and bilateral adnexal masses, though it is less likely to be associated with other Müllerian abnormalities. Almost all patients can be diagnosed by the above physical examination, and if necessary, perineal ultrasound and cystoscopy can assist confirming the diagnosis.

It is important to exclude other differential diagnosis such as MRKH syndrome, vaginal atresia, labial adhesion after infection, or radiotherapy. The first two disorders show normal vulvar vestibule and normal appearance of the labia majora and minora. Patients do not have normal menstrual flow, with (in vaginal atresia)/or without (in MRKH syndrome) periodic abdominal pain. The treatment of these vaginal anomalies is different from that of the labial fusion. Labial adhesion generally has a history of chronic inflammation of the vulva, vulval dysplasia, or a history of radiotherapy. Attention should be taken to have detailed history and physical examination.

3.3.2 Indication

If the condition is diagnosed, early surgical treatment is necessary.

3.3.3 Timing of Surgery

During puberty, patients with labial fusion usually present with abnormal menstrual blood flows or may also seek treatment because of difficulty at intercourse. Vulval surgery can expose the opening of the vagina, through which the menstrual blood can flow out normally after the surgery.

3.3.4 Contraindication

Before any surgery, it is important to identify the openings and positions of urethra, vagina, and rectum. If it confirms simple labia minora fusion, the following surgery can be performed. Otherwise, there can be risk of the urinary tract injury.

3.3.5 Preoperative Preparation

Preoperative pelvic ultrasound should be performed to define whether kidneys, ureters, and internal genital organs are normal, so as to exclude other congenital genital anomalies. If necessary, karyotyping and sex hormone and sex-related hormone or enzyme tests, such as 21-hydroxylase and cortisol levels, should be performed in order to confirm whether this vulval anomaly is due to clinical manifestations of other systemic endocrine disorders.

3.3.6 Surgical Procedure

Figures 3.6, 3.7, 3.8, 3.9, 3.10, and 3.11.

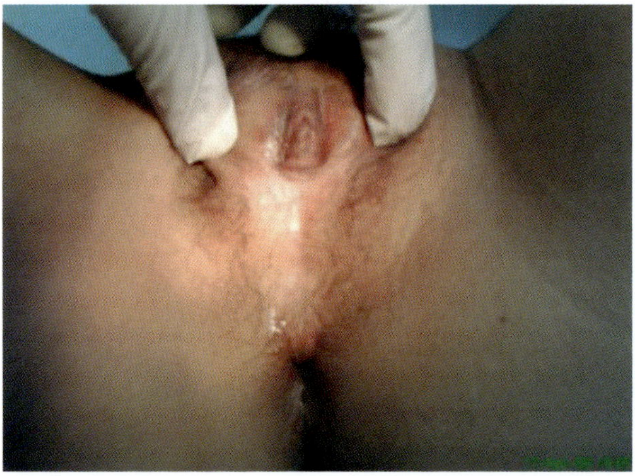

Fig. 3.6 The perineum should be adequately exposed and the vestibular structures defined. The perineum can be seen almost totally covered by perineal skin; there is a small opening below the clitoris without normal urethral and vaginal openings

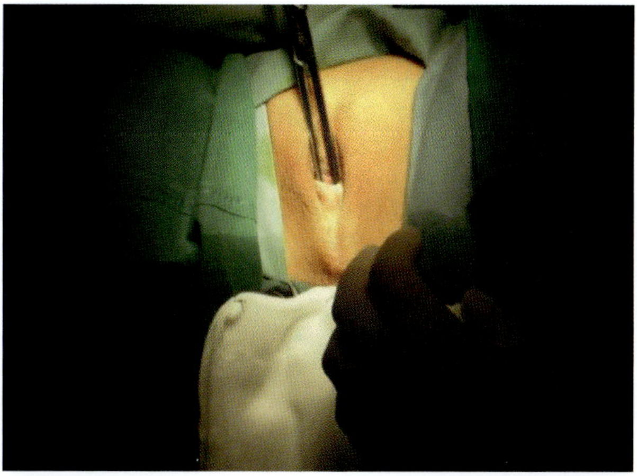

Fig. 3.7 An artery forceps is used to enlarge the above small opening. The artery forceps can then be inserted perpendicularly close to the perineal skin and run down towards the direction of the anus

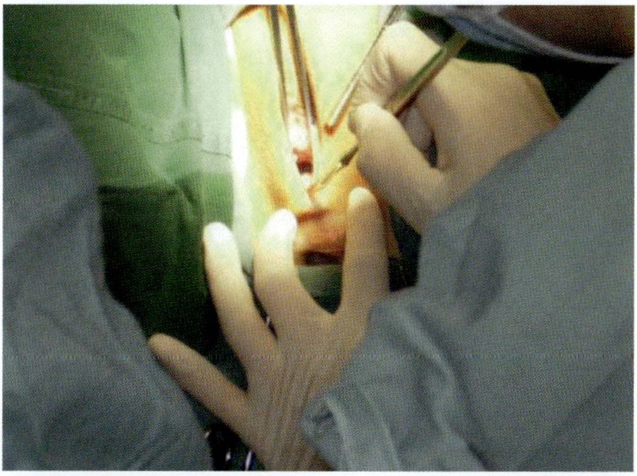

Fig. 3.8 Being guided by the artery forceps, the perineal skin can be incised down to the level of posterior vaginal wall, to expose the vaginal and urethral openings

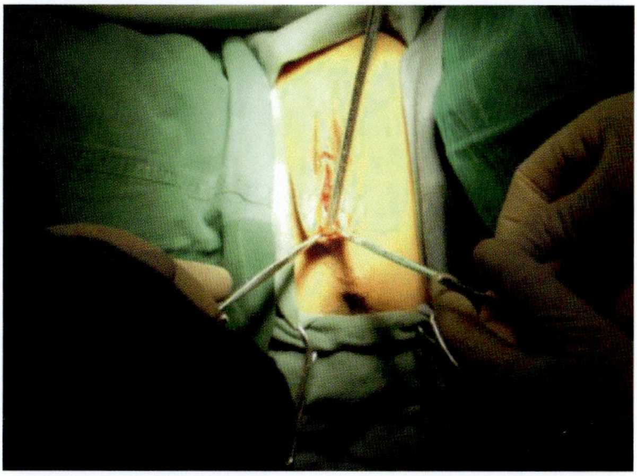

Fig. 3.9 Alice forceps are used to clamp the edges of incised perineal skins to provide hemostasis

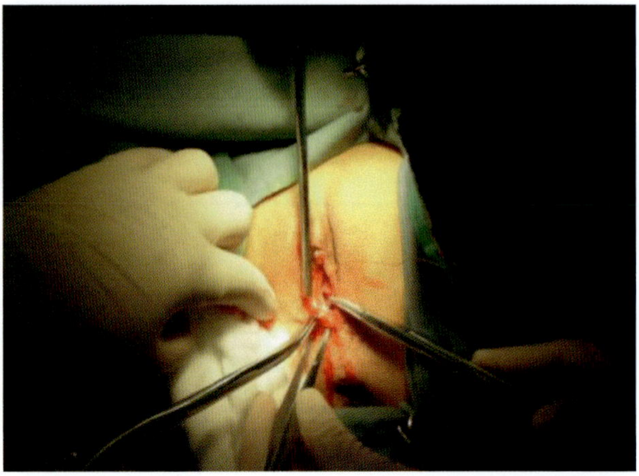

Fig. 3.10 The perineal wounds can then be sutured using 3/0 absorbable suture

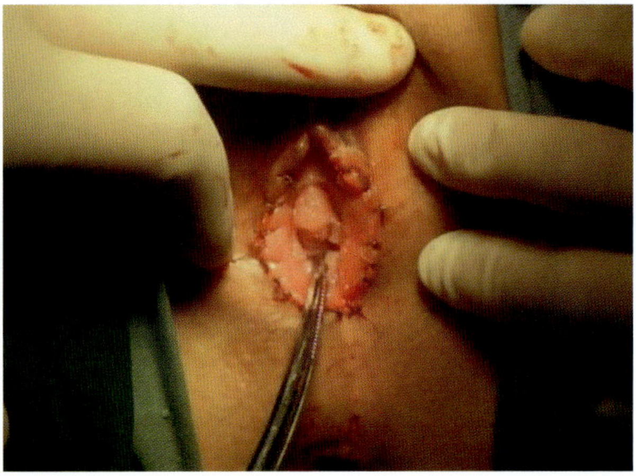

Fig. 3.11 After complete suturing, the labia minora will become the new vaginal opening, exposing the urethra and vagina

3.3.7 *Key Points of Surgery*

The success of this surgery is based on accurate diagnosis and better understanding of the anatomy of the vulva. It is important to adequately divide the fused perineal skin, to expose the vaginal and urethral openings.

References

1. Winderl LM, Silverman RK. Prenatal diagnosis of congenital imperforate hymen. Obstet Gynecol. 1995;85(5 Pt 2):857–60.
2. Capraro VJ, Dillon WP, Gallego MB. Microperforate hymen: a distinct clinical entity. Obstet Gynecol. 1974;44(6):903–5.
3. Sanfilippo AM, Mansuria SM. Microperforate hymen resulting in pelvic abscess. J Pediatr Adolesc Gynecol. 2006;19(2):95–8.
4. Stewart JF. Recurrent urinary tract infection in the female child secondary to a partial imperforate hymen. J Urol. 1970;103(3):353–6.
5. Shukunami K, Kaneshima M, Kurokawa T, Kubo M, Kotsuji F. Microperforate hymen at 27 years of age diagnosed with withdrawal bleeding and hysterofiberscopy. Arch Gynecol Obstet. 2000;264(1):49–50.
6. Guldberg R, Thybo S, Andersen B. Synechia vulva—an unusual cause of urinary symptoms in a 15-year-old girl. Acta Obstet Gynecol Scand. 2007;86(2):251–2. doi:10.1007/s00404-008-0598-3.
7. Puhl AG, Steiner E, Krämer WW, Weltzien A, Skala C, Passuello V, et al. Fetal urogenital sinus with consecutive hydrometrocolpos because of labial fusion prenatal diagnostic difficulties and postpartal therapeutic management. Fetal Diagn Ther. 2008;23(4):287–92. doi:10.1159/000123615.
8. Gul A, Yıldırım G, Gedıkbası A, Gungorduk K, Ceylan Y. Prenatal ultrasonographic features of persistent urogenital sinus with hydrometrocolpos and ascites. Arch Gynecol Obstet. 2008;278:493–6.

Chapter 4
Abnormal Development of the Vagina

Guangnan Luo, Hang Mei Jin, Li Bin, Huan-ying Wang, Xianghua Huang, Huimei Zhou, Lan Zhu, Jie Yang, Qiushi Wang, Xue Xiang, and Na Chen

4.1 Mayer-Rokitansky-Küster-Hauser (MRKH) Syndrome

4.1.1 Clinical Symptoms and Signs

Guangnan Luo

Congenital absence of vagina is often associated with no uterus or only a primordial uterus, while the fallopian tubes and ovaries develop normally. Patients will have secondary sexual characteristics of a normal female. Their karyotype is 46XX and is known as the Mayer-Rokitansky-Küster-Hauser syndrome (MRKH). The incidence of MRKH is 1/5000 to 1/4000. China is a country of very large population,

G. Luo
Department of Obstetrics and Gynecology, The Luohu Hospital of Shenzhen, Shenzhen, China

H.M. Jin
Department of Obstetrics, Affiliated Obstetrics and Gynecology Hospital, College of Medical Sciences, Zhejiang University, Hangzhou 310006, China

L. Bin • H.-y. Wang
Department of Obstetrics and Gynecology, An Zhen Hospital, Subsidiary of Capital Medical University, Beijing, China

X. Huang • Q. Wang
Department of Obstetrics and Gynecology, The Second Hospital of Hebei Medical University, Shijiazhuang, Hebei 050000, China

H. Zhou • L. Zhu (✉) • J. Yang • N. Chen
Department of Obstetrics and Gynecology, Peking Union Medical College Hospital, No. 1 Shuaifuyuan, Beijing 100730, P. R. China
e-mail: Zhu_julie@sina.com

X. Xiang
Department of Gynaecology and Obstetrics, The Second Affiliated Hospital, Medical School of Xi'an Jiaotong University, Xi'an, China

© Springer Science+Business Media Dordrecht 2015
L. Zhu et al. (eds.), *Atlas of Surgical Correction of Female Genital Malformation*, DOI 10.1007/978-94-017-7246-4_4

with an estimated 15 million patients suffering from MRKH. Many of them are living in rural areas and are not being diagnosed. For 11 years from 1986 to 1996, Tianjin City Centre Obstetrics and Gynecology Hospital had treated 109 patients of congenital absence of vagina, about 0.6 % of the total gynecologic inpatients in the same period. At the same time, from January 2003 to November 2013, the Shenzhen Luohu Hospital had treated 659 patients with congenital absence of vagina, accounting for 2.3 % of 28,364 gynecological inpatients in the same period.

4.1.1.1 Symptoms

1. Primary amenorrhea: Congenital absence of vagina is asymptomatic before puberty. They are discovered mainly in adolescence while they seek medical advice for primary amenorrhea.
2. Sexual difficulties: A small number of patients seek medical advice after their marriage because of difficulties in sexual intercourse. For some patients, the long-term upward pressure during sexual intercourse has created a vaginal hole, and they can even lead a normal marital life. Such a situation is more common in rural areas, just like the upward-pressure treatment method of vaginoplasty.
3. Cyclical abdominal pain: A small number of patients are with functional uteri, but following regular menstruations, they presented with cyclical abdominal pains. The abdominal pain may become very severe, affecting their lives and works, and warrant a timely hysterectomy.

4.1.1.2 Physical Signs

1. All patients with congenital absence of vagina (MRKH) have normal secondary female sexual characteristics.
2. Absence of the vagina: Patients will have normal external genitalia with normal vaginal vestibule and sometimes visible hymen, but without a vaginal opening (Fig. 4.1). When the vestibule is gently pressed with a finger, there will be various degrees of depressions from shallow to deep, called the vestibular depression (Fig. 4.2). Shallow ones can be 1–2 cm in depth and the deep ones up to 4–5 cm or even deeper.
3. Ovary: The ovarian development is normal, hence normal ovarian function with secondary sexual characteristics (Fig. 4.3).
4. Uterus: The uterus is mostly primordial with the size of a bean, situated at the medial ends of bilateral fallopian tubes (Fig. 4.3). A small number of uteri integrate in the midline to form a fibrous nodule posterior to the top of the bladder; sometimes it is referred as a trace of the uterus (Fig. 4.3). From both sides of the primordial uterus, there are fiber cords (Fig. 4.3). On the inner part on both cords, traces of sacral ligaments often are seen (Fig. 4.3). A small number of patients may even have a functional uterus, appearing as a solid spherical uterus but without the cervix and uterine cavity (Figs. 4.4 and 4.5), or with hypoplastic cervix and small uterine cavity. Sometimes, it leads to pelvic endometriosis, such as chocolate cysts (Fig. 4.6). The primordial uterus can also develop uterine fibroids (Fig. 4.7).
5. Other associated anomalies: A few patients with congenital absence of vagina may be associated with urinary tract anomalies. Common cases include the absence of kidney on one side, ectopic kidney, or pelvic kidney. Other patients may have associated spinal deformity. Common cases include lumbarization of first sacral spine, spina bifida, sacral recessive cleft, and vertebral fusion. If there are also abnormal secondary sexual characteristics and abnormal external genitalia, consideration should be given to chromosome abnormality or hermaphroditism.

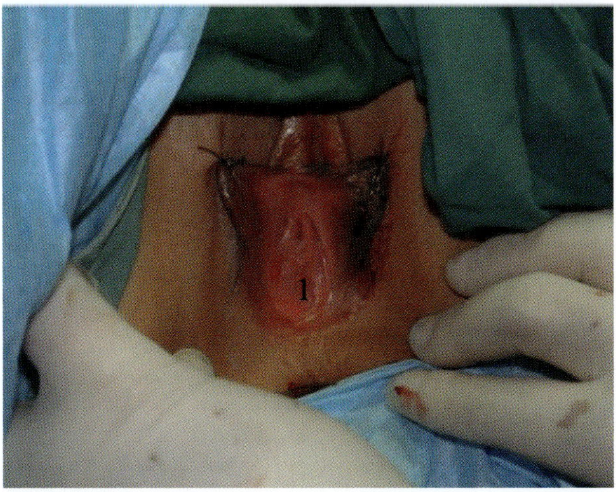

Fig. 4.1 The vulva of a patient with congenital absence of vagina. *1* Vestibule

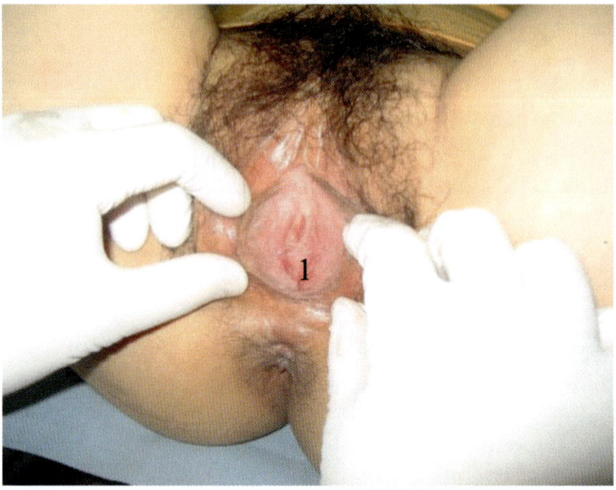

Fig. 4.2 Vestibular depression. *1* Vestibular depression

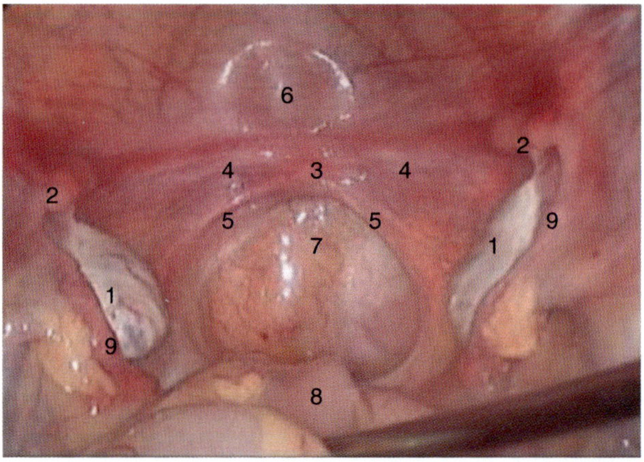

Fig. 4.3 Pelvic cavity of a patient with congenital absence of vagina. *1* Ovary, *2* primordial uterus, *3* trace of the uterus, *4* fibrous cord, *5* traces of the sacral ligament, *6* bladder, *7* pouch of Douglas, *8* rectum, *9* fallopian tubes

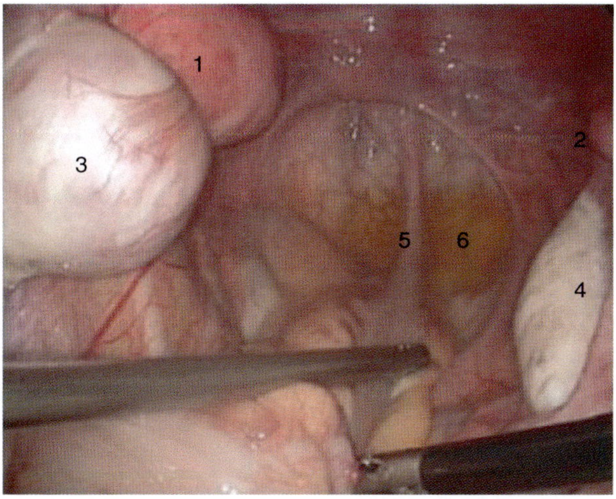

Fig. 4.4 Pelvic cavity of a functional primordial uterus. *1* Left functional primordial uterus, *2* right nonfunctional primordial uterus, *3* left chocolate cyst, *4* right ovary, *5* rectum, *6* pouch of Douglas

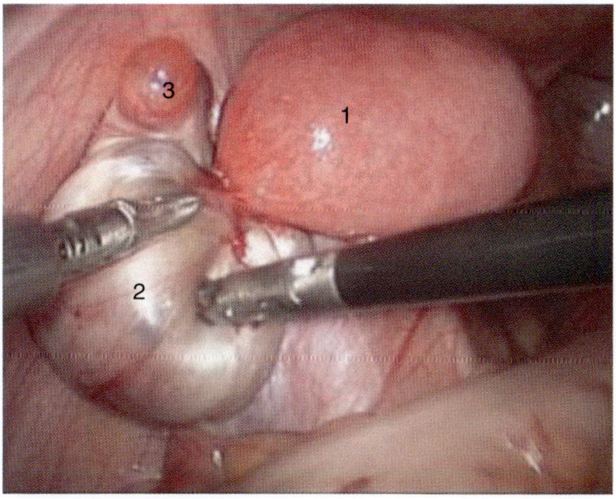

Fig. 4.5 Functional uterus. *1* Left functional primordial uterus, *2* left chocolate cyst, *3* follicular cyst

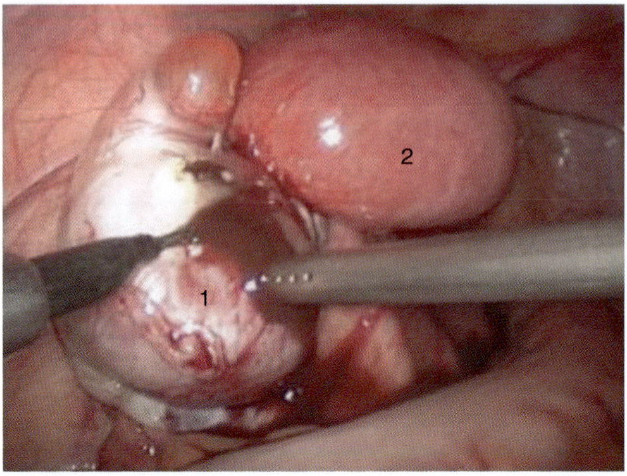

Fig. 4.6 Functional uterus with chocolate cyst, associated with severe cyclical abdominal pain. *1* Left ovarian chocolate cyst, *2* left functional uterus

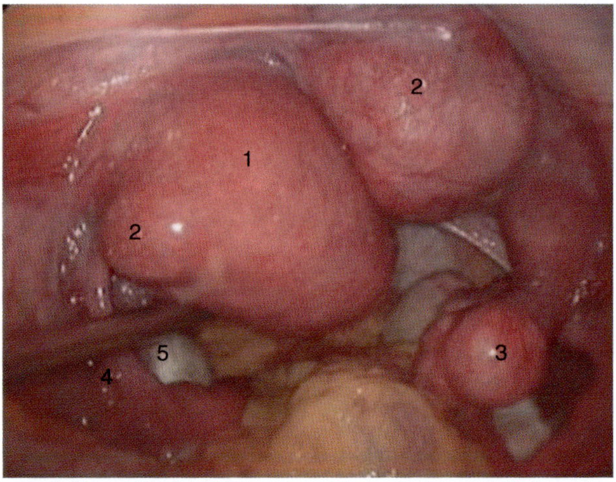

Fig. 4.7 Functional uterus with fibroid. *1* left functional uterus, *2* uterine fibroid, *3* right primodial uterus, *4* left fallopian tube, *5* left ovary

4.1.2 *Diagnosis and Investigations*

The diagnosis is not difficult. In addition to the clinical history and physical signs, there are many useful investigations.

4.1.2.1 Gynecological Examination

Vestibular depression test (or depth of vestibular impression): After observing the vulval appearance, the vaginal vestibule is gently pressed with a gloved index finger lubricated with paraffin oil. With gradually increasing pressure, the depth of vestibular depression can be determined (Figs. 4.8, 4.9, and 4.10). Some depression can be over 5–6 cm in depth. This vestibular depression test is useful to select the type of surgical operations for this condition.

4.1.2.2 Rectal (PR) Examination

PR examination can determine whether there is a uterus, its size, and any tenderness on palpation. It is generally difficult to palpate an absent uterus or small primordial uteri on both sides of the pelvis. Only if it is a uterine remnant at the back behind the top of the bladder, then a small nodular mass can be palpable (Fig. 4.3). If the uterus is enlarged and painful, it is most likely a functional uterus with retained blood (Figs. 4.6 and 4.7).

4.1.2.3 Ultrasound Examination

This is the most important and simple examination to determine whether there is a vaginal gas line, the size of uteri, ovaries, and the existence and locations of the kidneys.

4.1.2.4 Other Examinations

A few patients may require X-ray imaging or CT-scan examinations, in order to detect any urinary tract abnormality or spinal deformity.

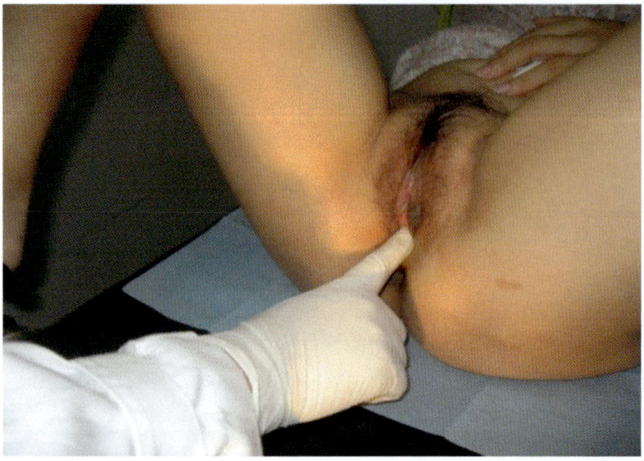

Fig. 4.8 Vestibular depression test. The vulval vestibule is pressed with gloved index finger

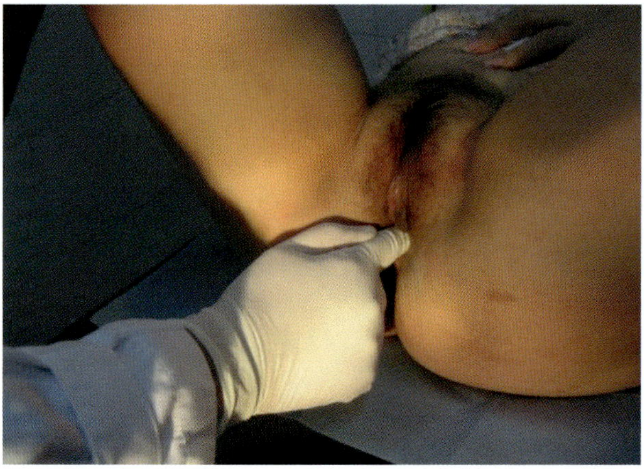

Fig. 4.9 The deepest point is reached by the finger, and the depth of depression is marked by the thumb

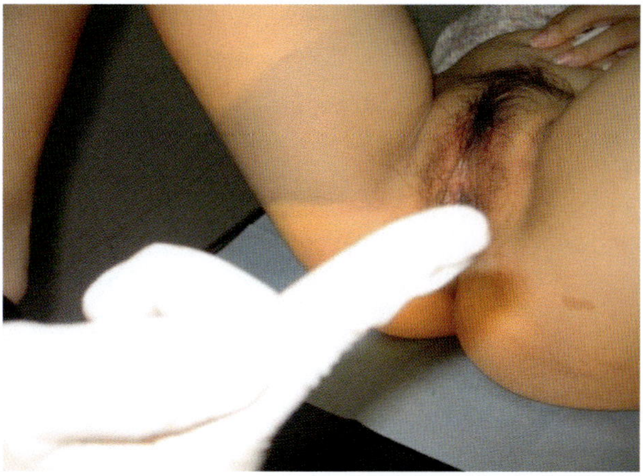

Fig. 4.10 The depth of vestibular depression is the distance from the fingertip to the marking thumb

4.1.3 Timing of Surgery

For patients with congenital absence of vagina (MRKH), operation is generally performed for adults after 18 years of age. For those who have periodic abdominal pain caused by a functional bleeding uterus, surgery should be performed as soon as possible to relieve the symptoms.

Currently, many doctors tell their patients with congenital absence of vagina to have surgery 2–3 months before marriage. This is inappropriate advice on the timing of surgery. It is because a woman without a vagina will have serious worry and concern about having a love affair with a man. This will lead to psychological barrier, and they will not dare to touch the men, hence inducing a sense of inferiority. They will abstain from the society and people. Some doctors are concerned with the stenosis and atrophy of the new vagina due to the lack of sex life. In fact, such concerns are unnecessary. A successful new vagina will not shrink. Even if not married, a vagina mold can often be used to expand the vagina to obtain satisfactory results.

4.1.4 Laparoscopic Peritoneal Vaginoplasty: Luo Hu Operation

Guangnan Luo

There are many surgical approaches for laparoscopic peritoneal vaginoplasty. This section highlights the "Luo Hu Operation" pioneered by Dr. Luo Guang Nan from the Affiliated Hospital of Shenzhen University. This laparoscopic-assisted peritoneal vaginoplasty – Luo Hu Operation – is characterized by its simplicity, easy to learn, and minimally invasive. The postoperative result is good, especially without the need to wear a vaginal mold for a long period.

4.1.4.1 Operative Indications

(a) Patients with congenital absence of vagina and uterus
(b) Patients with androgen insensitivity syndrome with vaginal anomalies

4.1.4.2 Contraindications

(a) Patients with severe pelvic adhesions
(b) Patients with male sex reassignment surgery to become a male

4.1.4.3 Preoperative Preparation

(a) Preoperative bowel preparations using low-residue diet and oral bowel antibiotic are recommended for 3 days before surgery, and enema is given in the previous night and the morning of surgery. It is to prepare for the situations when this surgical approach fails to complete, then it can be changed immediately to the sigmoid colon or ileum vaginoplasty.
(b) Special surgical instruments

   1. "Luo Hu style" vaginal dilators (for use in surgery): A total of six vaginal dilators should be available. They are about 20–25 cm in length with blunt conical tips. Their diameters ranged from small to large as No. 1–2.2 cm, No. 2–2.5 cm, No. 3–2.8 cm, No. 4–3.0 cm, No. 5–3.3 cm, and No. 6–3.5 cm, respectively (Fig. 4.11).

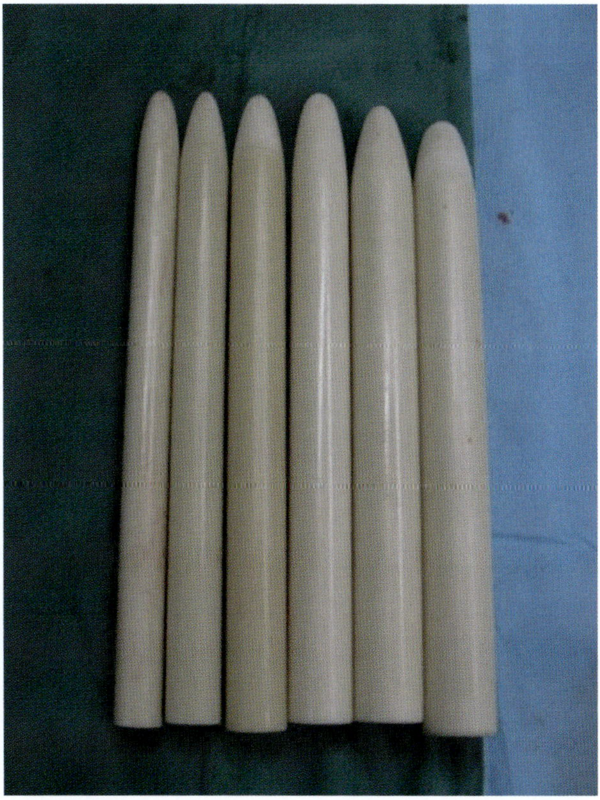

Fig. 4.11 Luo Hu style vaginal dilators

2. A No. 0 Prolene (Ethicon Prolene 8418) nonabsorbable suture.
3. An extracorporeal knot pusher.
4. Injection fluid: 200–300 ml of normal saline with six units Pitressin and 1 mg Epinephrine for lifting pelvic peritoneum by distension.
5. Homemade disposable vaginal mold: Take a 5 ml size syringe jacket, cut its ends, covering it with Vaseline gauze to about a thumb size in thickness. The new mold is further coated with three layers of condoms and ligated with No. 4 silk suture at its tail. After that, the excess condom material is cut off, leaving a short tail (Fig. 4.12).

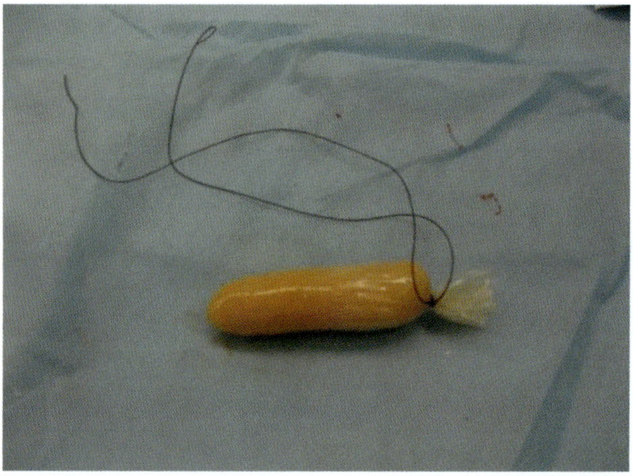

Fig. 4.12 Homemade disposable vaginal mold

4.1.4.4 Surgical Techniques

Diagrams of Luo Hu Operation (Figs. 4.13, 4.14, 4.15, 4.16, 4.17, 4.18, 4.19, 4.20, 4.21, and 4.22)

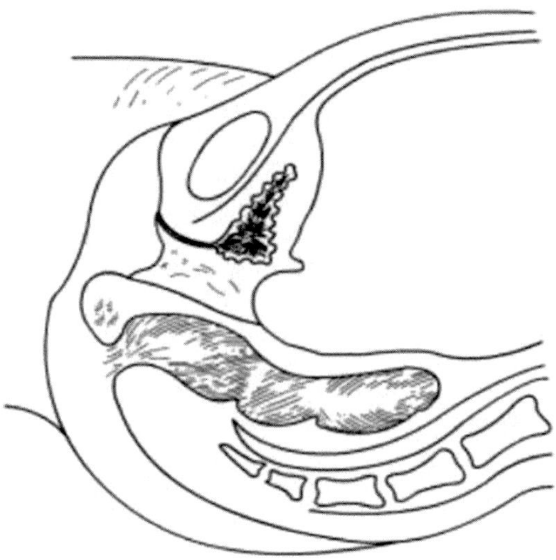

Fig. 4.13 Sagittal view of the pelvis in a patient with congenital absence of vagina and uterus

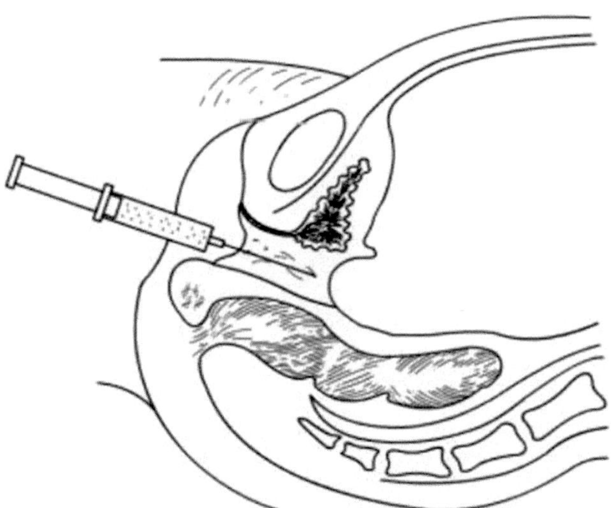

Fig. 4.14 Inject normal saline at the pelvic extraperitoneal space to create a water cushion between the bladder and rectum

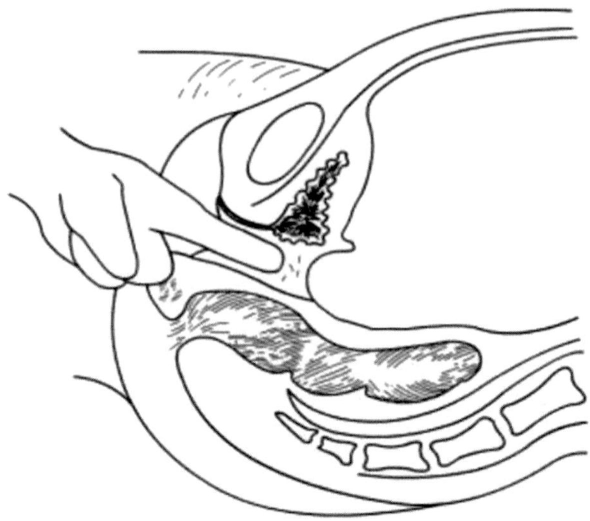

Fig. 4.15 Creating a vaginal tunnel with one or two index fingers of both hands

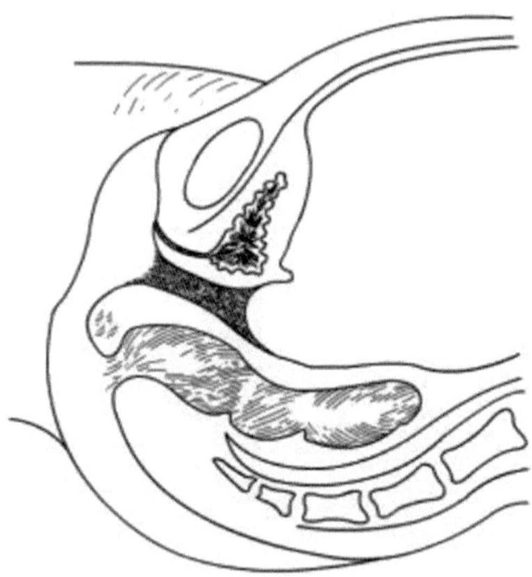

Fig. 4.16 A vaginal tunnel is created by pressure, stretching, and separating by fingers

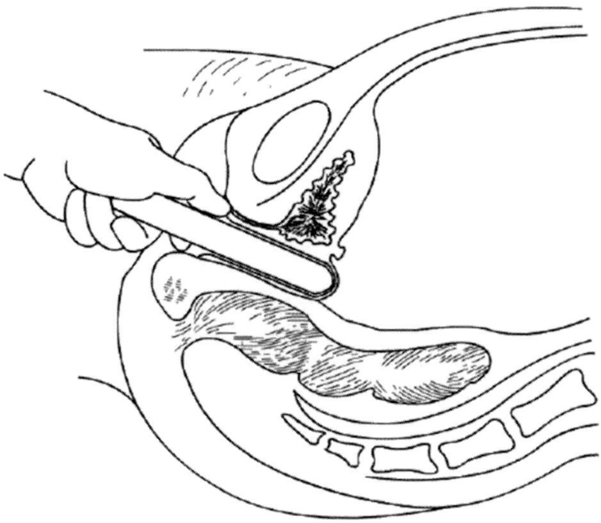

Fig. 4.17 A small-sized vaginal dilator is inserted into the tunnel, to push up the pelvic peritoneum behind the bladder

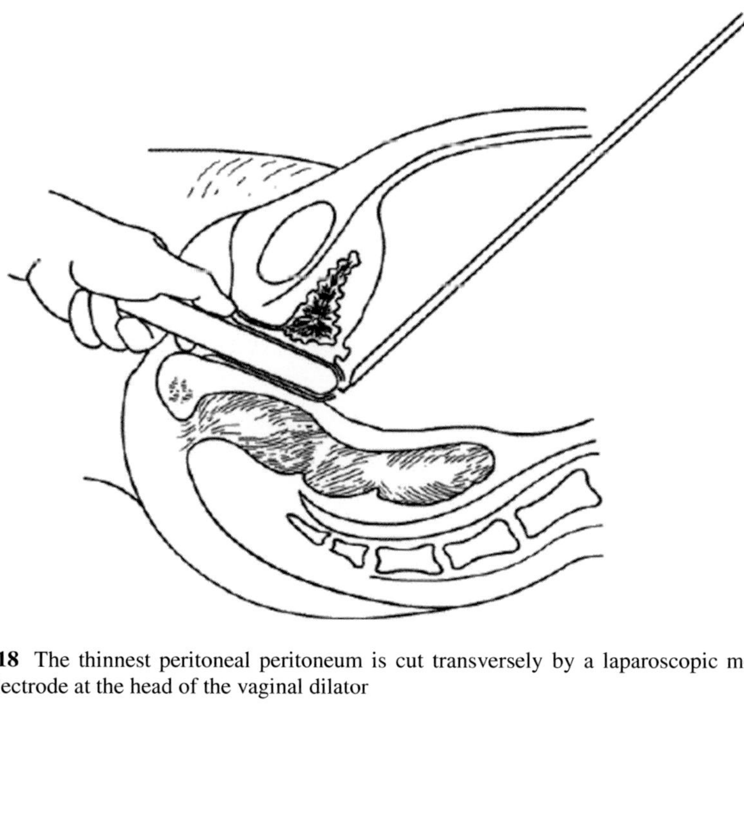

Fig. 4.18 The thinnest peritoneal peritoneum is cut transversely by a laparoscopic monopolar hook electrode at the head of the vaginal dilator

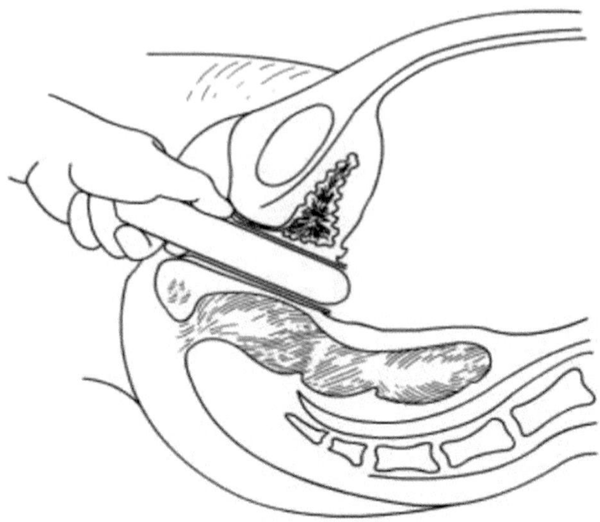

Fig. 4.19 The new vaginal tunnel is enlarged with small- to large-sized vaginal dilators, and the peritoneal opening is further cut open

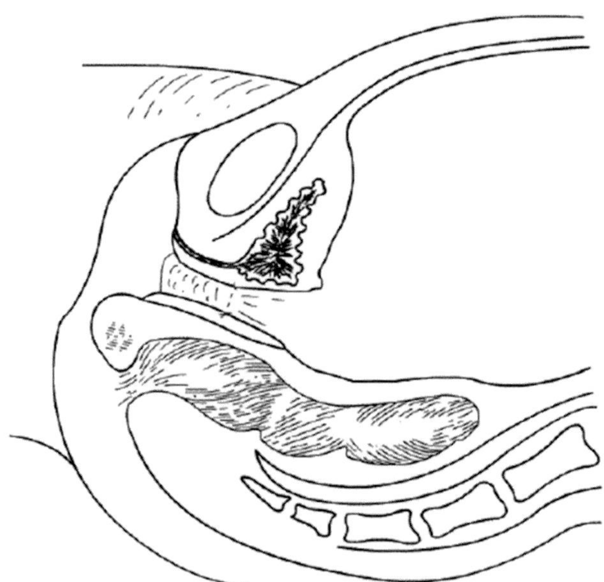

Fig. 4.20 The edge of the pelvic peritoneum is now pulled down to the vaginal opening and stitched to the vaginal mucosa at the vestibule. The pelvic peritoneum is now completely covering the vaginal tunnel

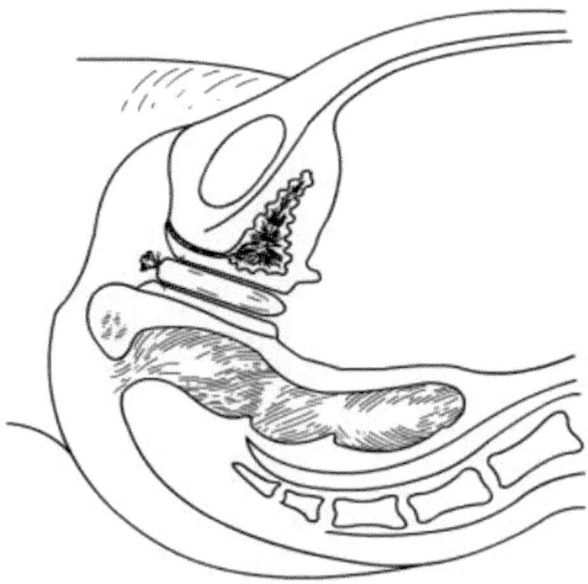

Fig. 4.21 A vaginal mold is inserted into the new vaginal tunnel

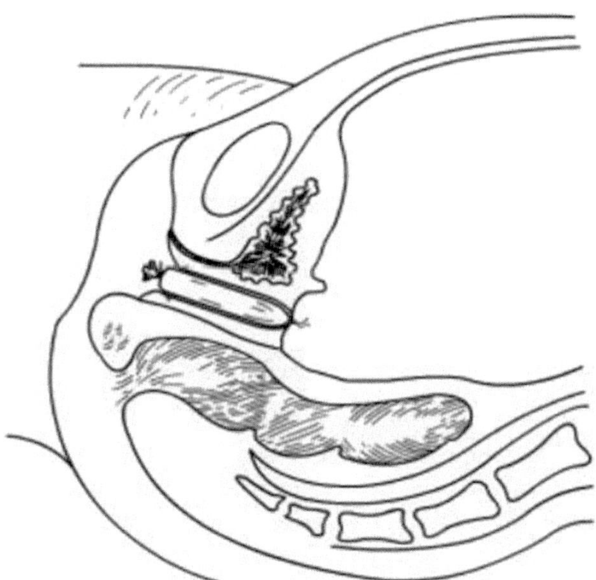

Fig. 4.22 The peritoneal opening in the pelvis is now closed, and a new vagina has been created

4.1.4.5 Surgical Procedures

Position

Patient is in a lithotomy position. Operation is performed under general anesthesia.

Insertion of a Foley Catheter

Bladder is catheterized emptied with an indwelling catheter F16 or F18. A large-sized catheter should be chosen in order to guide the creation of the vaginal tunnel serving as a direction marker, to avoid damage to the urethra.

Laparoscopic Examination of the Pelvic Cavity

A 10 mm size laparoscope is inserted into the peritoneal cavity via the umbilicus. Two 5 mm operating trocars and cannulas are inserted on both lower abdominal quadrants to examine the pelvic cavity, to observe and evaluate the pelvic peritoneum, bilateral adnexa, and the location and size of the primordial uterus.

Creation of an Extraperitoneal Water Cushion

An epidural needle is used to puncture into the center of the vaginal vestibule (Fig. 4.23), pass through the gap between the urethra and bladder in front, and rectum behind directly to the extraperitoneal space over the pouch of Douglas. The needle tip can be seen, under the laparoscope, just below the peritoneal surface, but care is taken not to puncture the peritoneum (Figs. 4.24 and 4.25). Saline with vasopressin and adrenaline is injected into the extraperitoneal space to form a large water cushion (Fig. 4.26). A successful water cushion will push up the pelvic peritoneum which appears white in color (Fig. 4.27), and hence separating and pushing up the pelvic peritoneum from the pelvic floor. The water cushion will also push back the rectal wall, to make it easier to create a channel for the new vagina and prevent the rectal wall from injury, as well as to reduce bleeding during this procedure (Fig. 4.28). The needle is slowly withdrawn while injecting more saline up to a total of 200–300 ml to fill up the space between the urethra, the bladder, and the rectum to facilitate the next step of making a tunnel.

The Creation of a Vaginal Tunnel

At the punctured hole in the center of the vaginal vestibule, a medium-sized curved forceps is used to puncture through the mucosal membrane, then in a direction parallel to the urethra, the tissue up to 3–4 cm is stretched opened (Figs. 4.29 and 4.30).

Then an index finger is inserted into the space, bluntly separating the tissue in the direction parallel to the Foley catheter and creating a tunnel in the space among the urethra, the bladder, and the rectum (Figs. 4.31, 4.32, and 4.33). The smallest-sized vaginal dilator is then inserted into the newly created tunnel and is pushed further in toward the pelvic floor (Fig. 4.34). Under the laparoscope, the head of the vaginal dilator can be seen behind the bladder pushing toward the pelvic peritoneum. A pair of laparoscopic graspers can be used to grip the transverse fibrous cords at the bottom of the bladder and push the bladder up and forward so that the peritoneum of the pouch of Douglas between the rectum and the bladder can be seen firmly pressed against the head of the vaginal dilator (Fig. 4.35).

A monopolar hook electrode is used to incise the peritoneum transversely at the thinnest spot at the head of the vaginal dilator (Fig. 4.36), then push the dilator toward the peritoneal incision to expand it (Fig. 4.37). The dilators are progressively changed (Fig. 4.38) from small to large size (No. 1 to No. 6) (Figs. 4.39 and 4.40) to expand the tunnel (Figs. 4.41 and 4.42).

A 3/0 absorbable suture is now passed into the pelvic cavity through the vaginal opening (Fig. 4.43). Under the laparoscopic vision, the incised peritoneal edges are marked with sutures at 12, 3, 6, and 9 o'clock positions, respectively. The needles with their sutures are then pulled out of the vaginal opening at the vestibule. These sutures are then sutured with the mucous membrane of the vaginal vestibule at corresponding 12, 3, 6, and 9 o'clock positions. Now the entire vaginal tunnel is covered with the peritoneal membrane (Figs. 4.44, 4.45, 4.46, 4.47, 4.48, 4.49, 4.50, 4.51, 4.52, 4.53, 4.54, 4.55, 4.56, and 4.57). A nonabsorbable 1/0 Prolene is passed into the pelvic cavity through the vagina and is used to close the pelvic floor (Fig. 4.58) for later closure of the peritoneum. A homemade vagina mold (Fig. 4.12) is inserted into the vagina (Fig. 4.59) reaching the cutting edge of the tunnel at the pelvic floor (Fig. 4.60) to prevent adhesion, provide hemostasis, and maintain the space of the tunnel. The vaginal opening is then sutured temporarily to hold the mold inside the vagina (Figs. 4.61 and 4.62).

Suturing the Pelvic Floor

Under the laparoscopic vision, the 1/0 nonabsorbable Prolene, which has purposely left in the pelvic cavity in the last step, is now picked up and used to close the pelvic floor peritoneum using a purse-string suture over the inner tunnel above the vaginal mold (Fig. 4.63). Six extracorporeal knots are tied from outside and pushed down into the peritoneal cavity, closing the pelvic peritoneal opening securely. Although the newly formed pelvic floor may have gaps in the peritoneum, no further suturing is needed. When the pneumoperitoneum is released, the gaps will disappear, followed by reperitonealization to form a closed pelvic floor 10 days after surgery (Figs. 4.64, 4.65, 4.66, and 4.67).

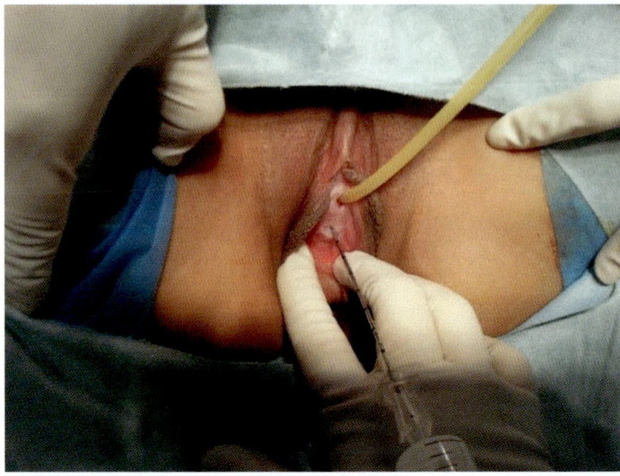

Fig. 4.23 A long epidural needle with 20 ml syringe filled with normal saline is inserted into the middle of the vaginal vestibule

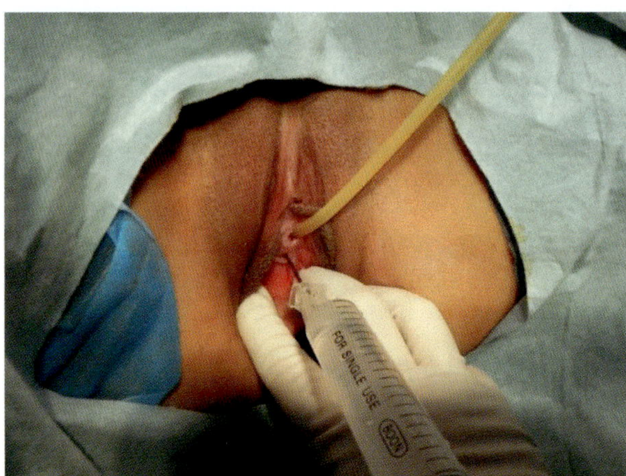

Fig. 4.24 The needle is advancing into the tissue in a direction parallel to the urinary catheter up to 3–4 cm

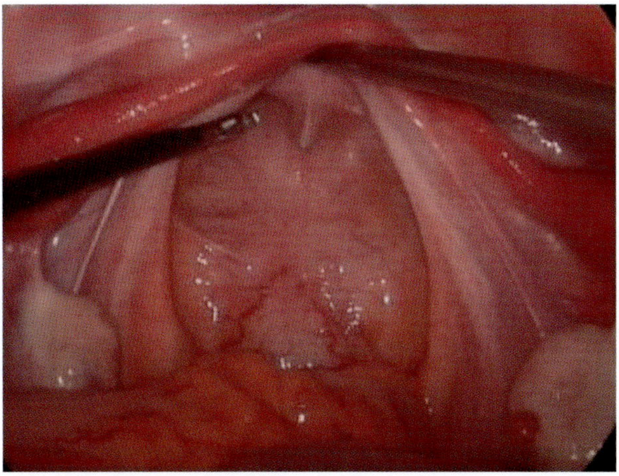

Fig. 4.25 Under laparoscopy, the needle is inserted into the space between the bladder and the rectum up to the peritoneum of the pouch of Douglas. It is important not to puncture the peritoneum

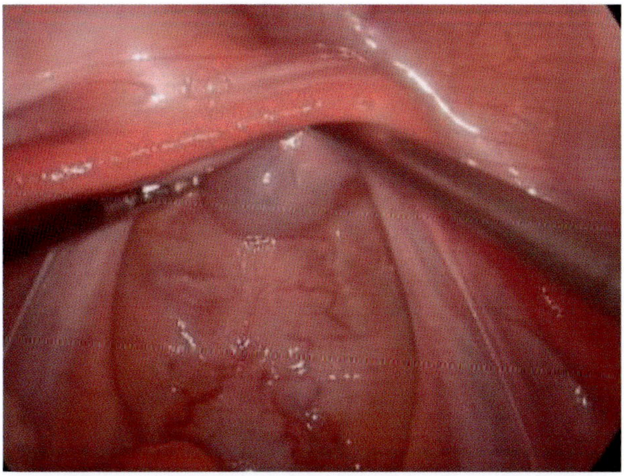

Fig. 4.26 Normal saline is injected underneath the pelvic peritoneum, to form a white and semi-transparent water cushion

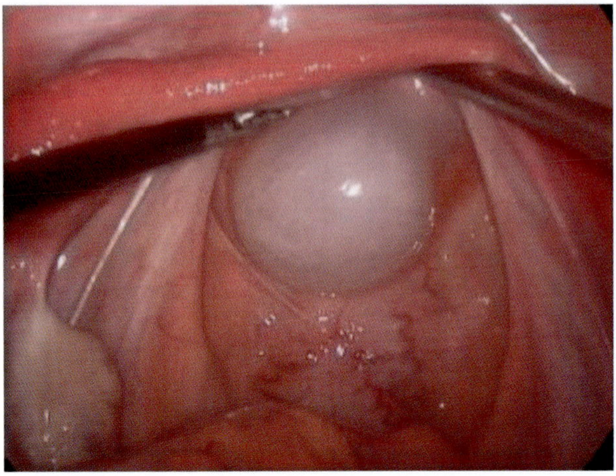

Fig. 4.27 Normal saline is slowly injected and the water cushion is getting bigger

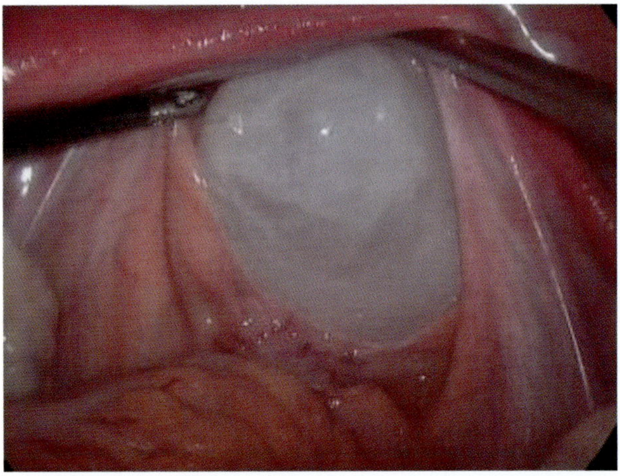

Fig. 4.28 The peritoneal membrane appears milky white in color, indicating that it has separated from the pelvic floor, the bladder, and the anterior wall of the rectum

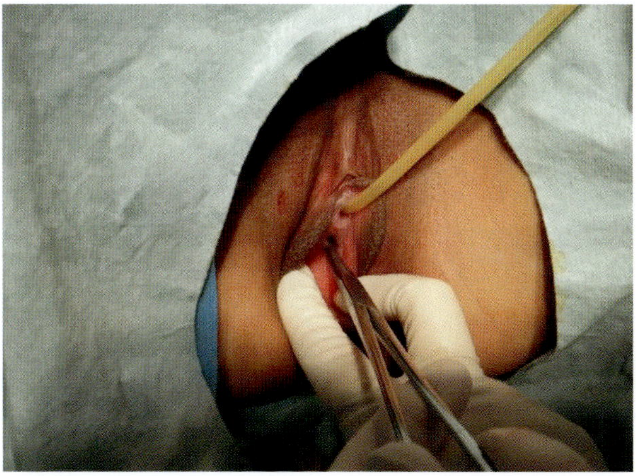

Fig. 4.29 The mucosa of the vaginal vestibule is punctured by inserting a medium or large curved forceps in order to penetrate and separate the tissue

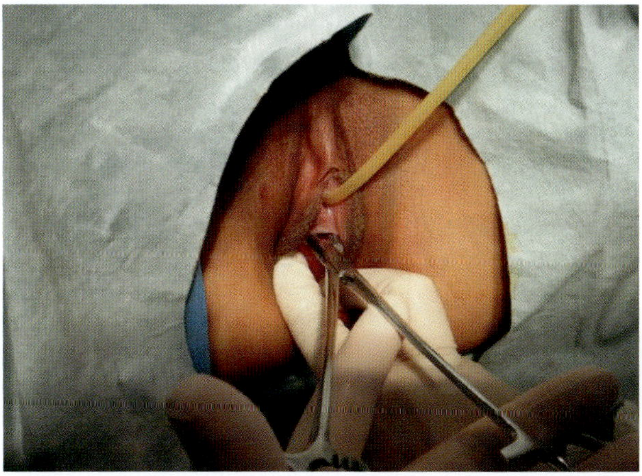

Fig. 4.30 After advancing 3–4 cm in depth, the curved forceps is to open and to separate the intervening tissue

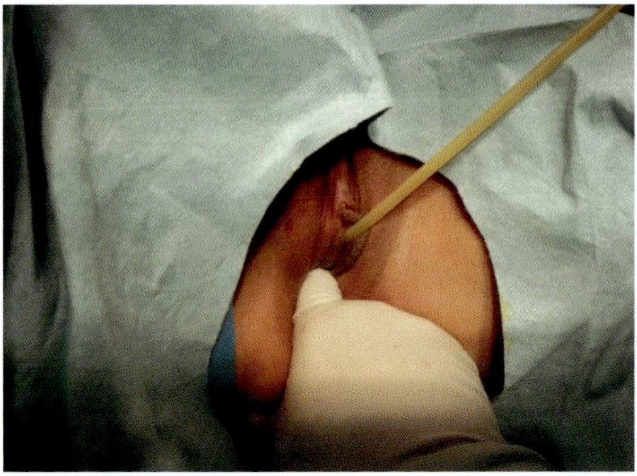

Fig. 4.31 An index finger is inserted into the tissue space to make further separation of the tissue

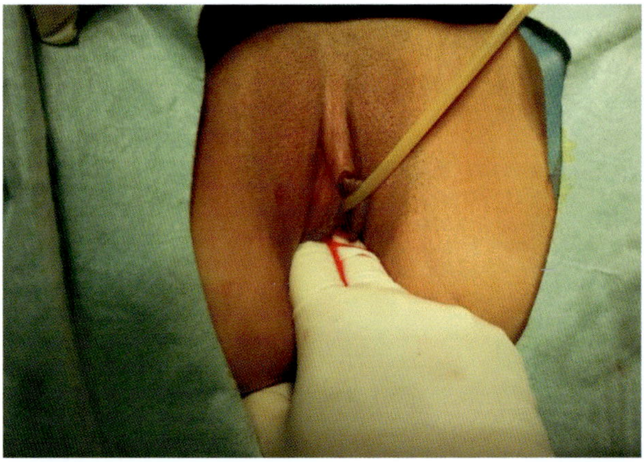

Fig. 4.32 Index and middle fingers are used to separate digitally the tissue until they reach the water cushion and pelvic peritoneum overlying it. The vaginal tunnel is now created

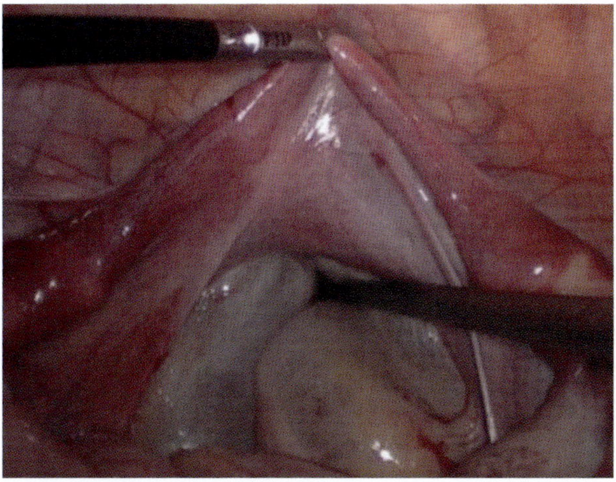

Fig. 4.33 Under the guide of the laparoscopy, an index finger will further separate the peritoneal membrane along the sides of a vaginal guide rod

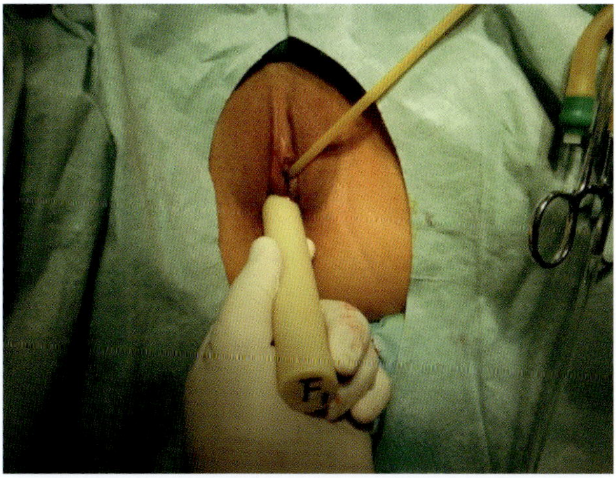

Fig. 4.34 The smallest vaginal dilator is inserted into the vaginal tunnel

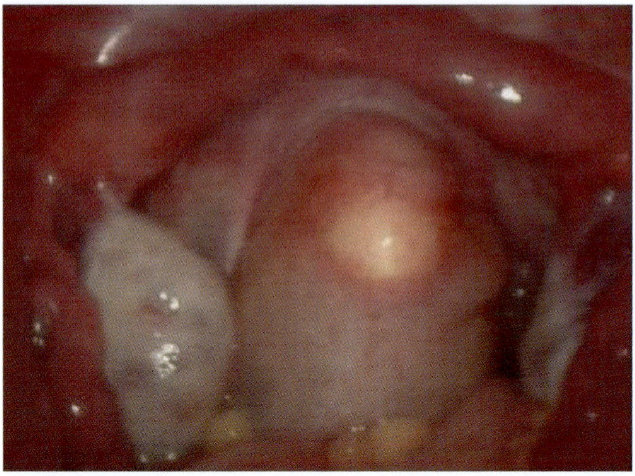

Fig. 4.35 A vaginal dilator now elevates the pelvic peritoneum which is very thin and white in color, suggesting that the anterior wall of the rectum is not close by, and is probably separated from the peritoneum

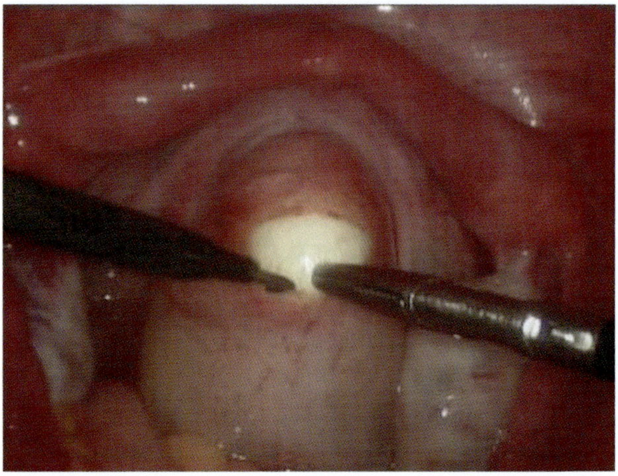

Fig. 4.36 A monopolar hook electrode or electrocautery is used to incise the peritoneal membrane at the head of the vaginal dilator

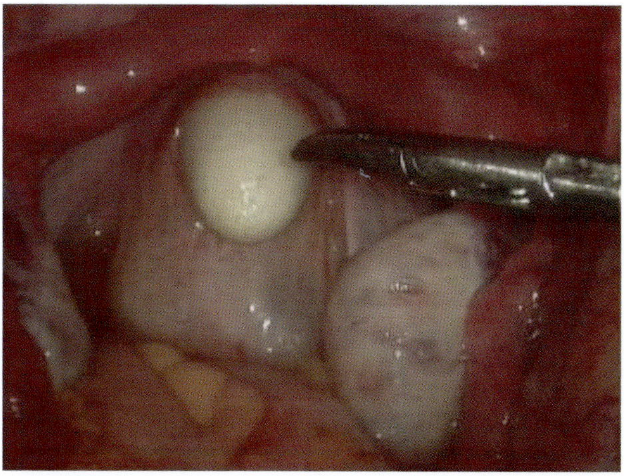

Fig. 4.37 A vaginal dilator is inserted through the peritoneal wound to expand the incision opening

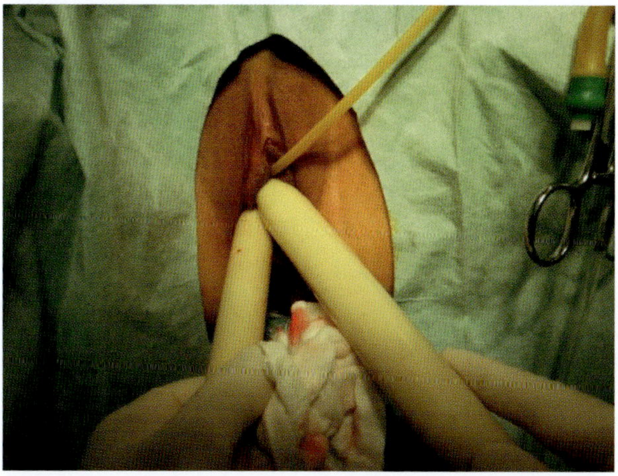

Fig. 4.38 Vaginal dilator is changed from small to large size to expand the vaginal tunnel and incision opening

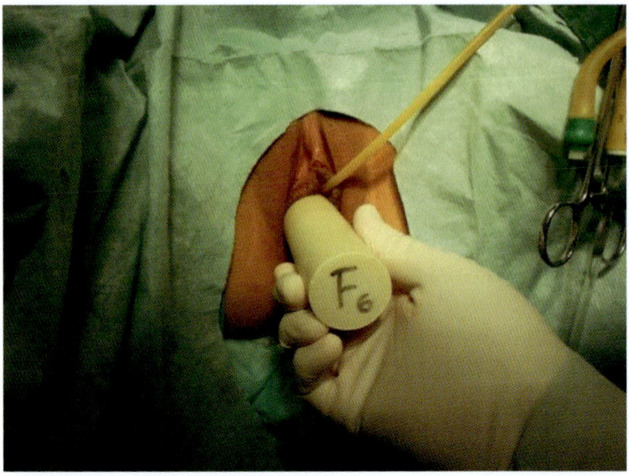

Fig. 4.39 The vaginal dilator is changed progressively from No. 1, No. 2, etc. till the largest No. 6 dilator was inserted into the vaginal tunnel

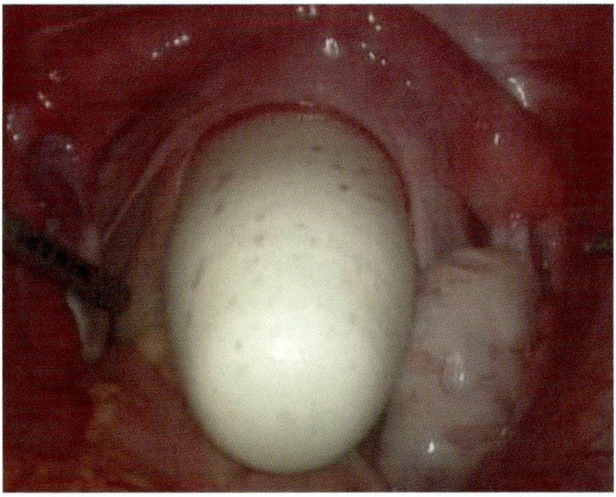

Fig. 4.40 Laparoscopic view of the largest No. 6 vaginal dilator at the peritoneal opening

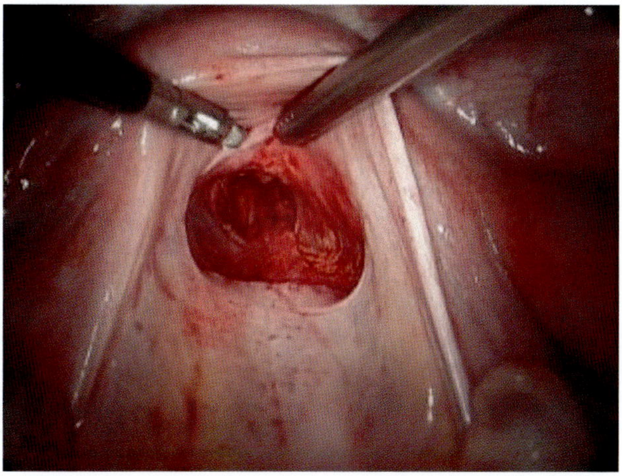

Fig. 4.41 The new vagina is created at the pouch of Douglas. There is minimal bleeding

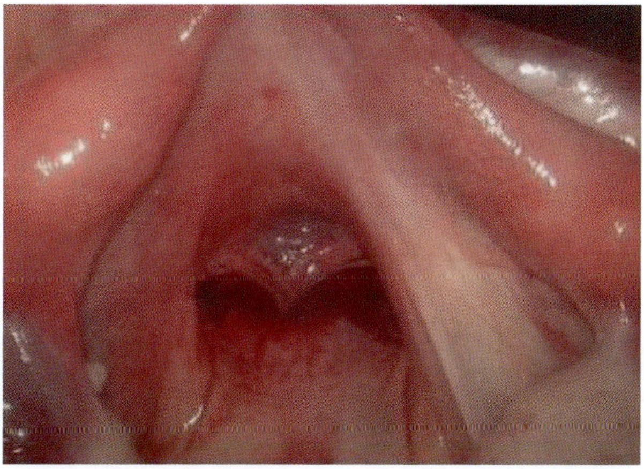

Fig. 4.42 The separated peritoneum is seen hanging over the pelvic peritoneal opening

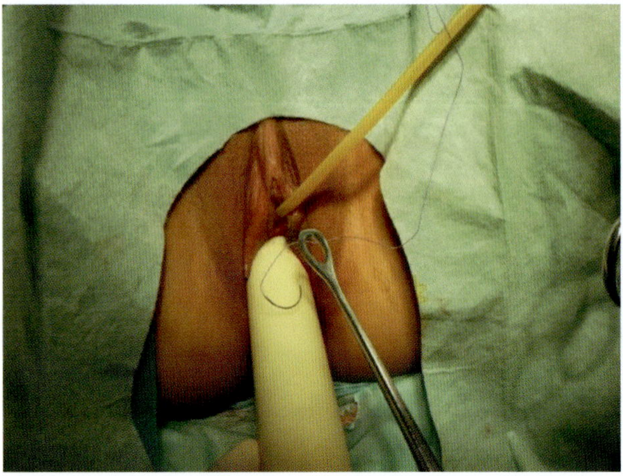

Fig. 4.43 Four 3/0 Vicryl sutures are introduced into the pelvic cavity via the vaginal tunnel, leaving the ends of these sutures outside the vaginal opening

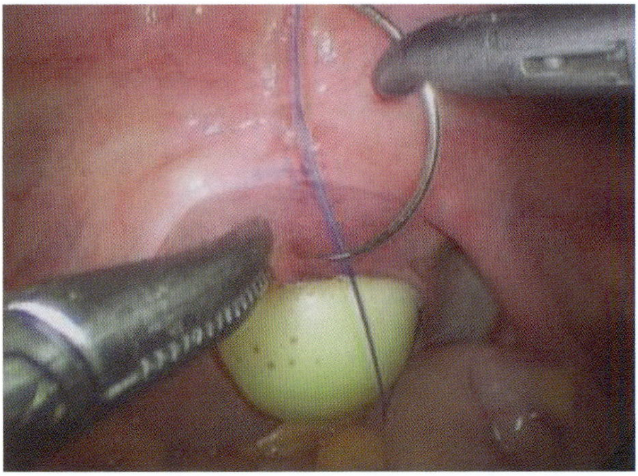

Fig. 4.44 The pelvic peritoneum at 12 o'clock position is marked and sutured at the inner vaginal opening

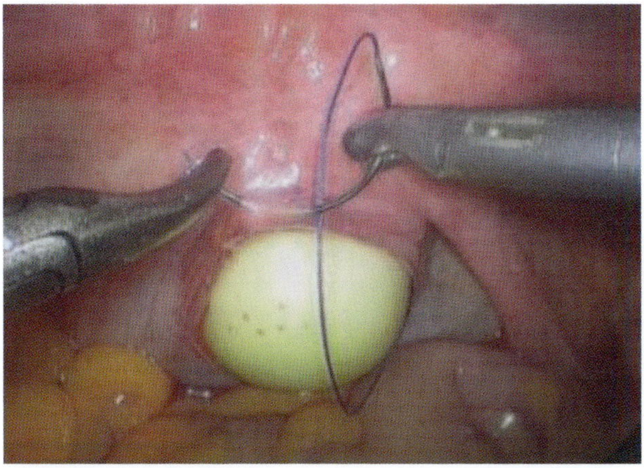

Fig. 4.45 The needle passes through the peritoneum

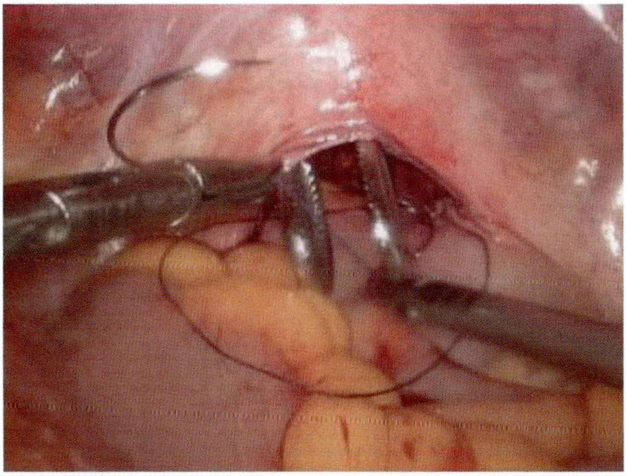

Fig. 4.46 A ring forceps is inserted through the vaginal tunnel to pick up the suture

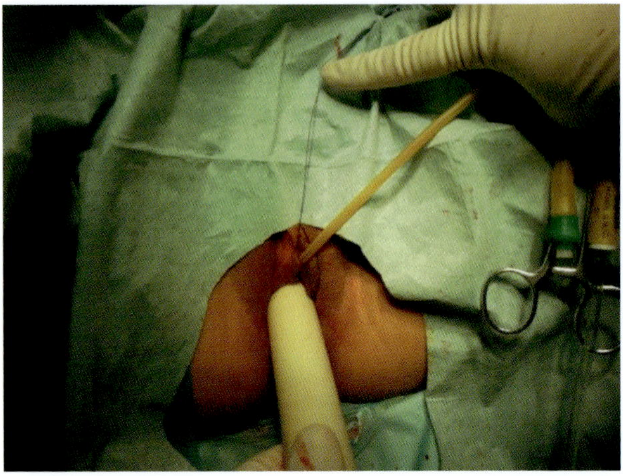

Fig. 4.47 The suture is pulled out of the vaginal opening and anchored at the corresponding 12 o'clock position of the vaginal vestibule

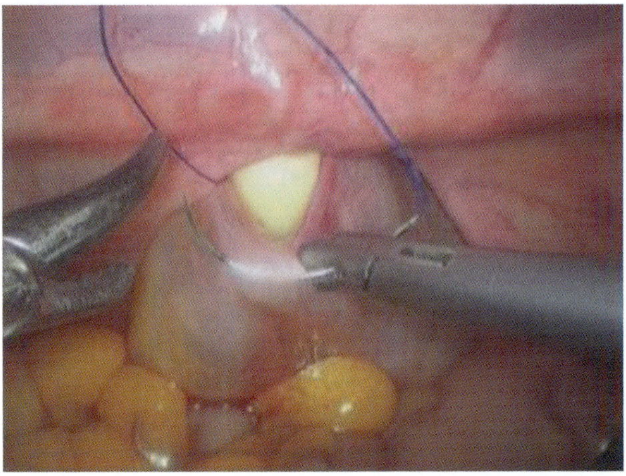

Fig. 4.48 Similarly, another suture is inserted to pick up the peritoneal membrane at the 6 o'clock by suturing it

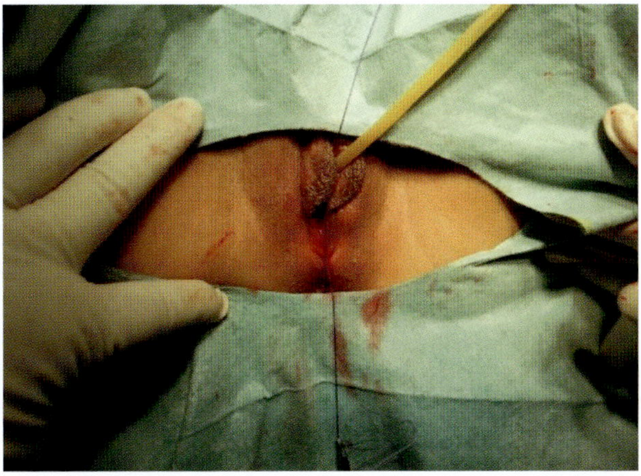

Fig. 4.49 Both sutures are anchored at the 12 o'clock and 6 o'clock positions of the vaginal opening

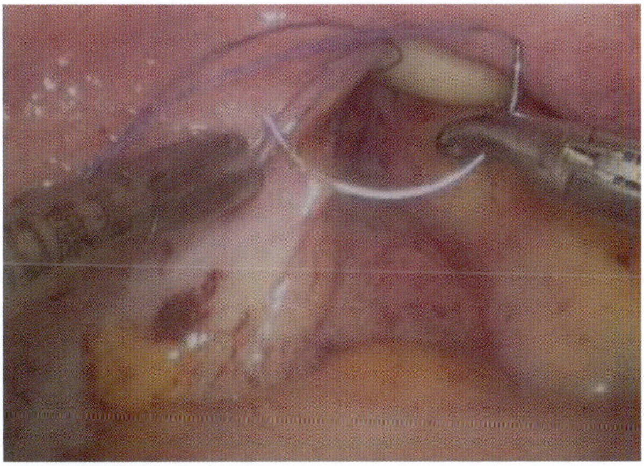

Fig. 4.50 Similar procedure is to pick up the left peritoneum edge

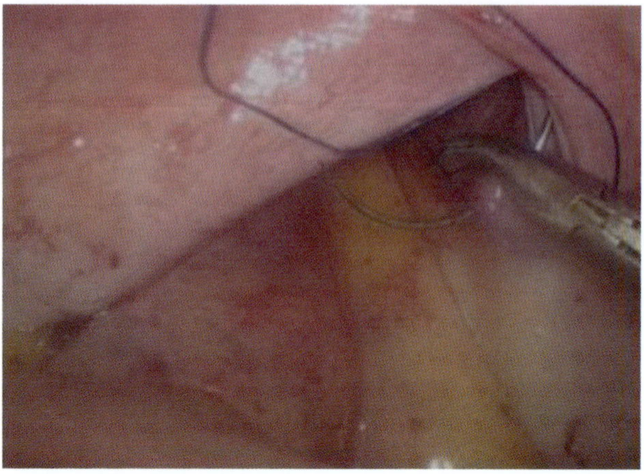

Fig. 4.51 Same to the right peritoneum edge

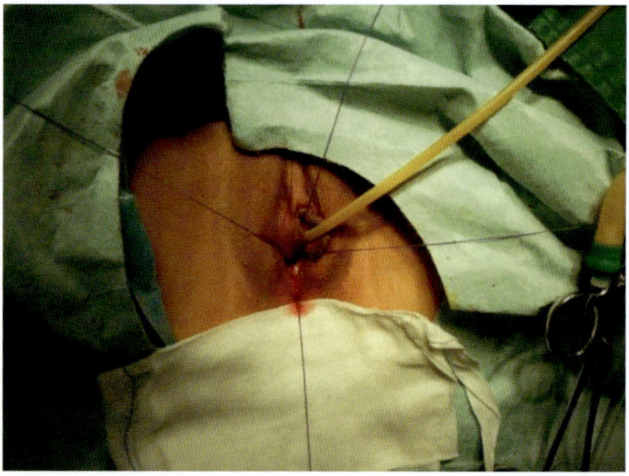

Fig. 4.52 These sutures are anchored at the corresponding 12, 3, 6, and 9 o'clock positions at the vaginal opening

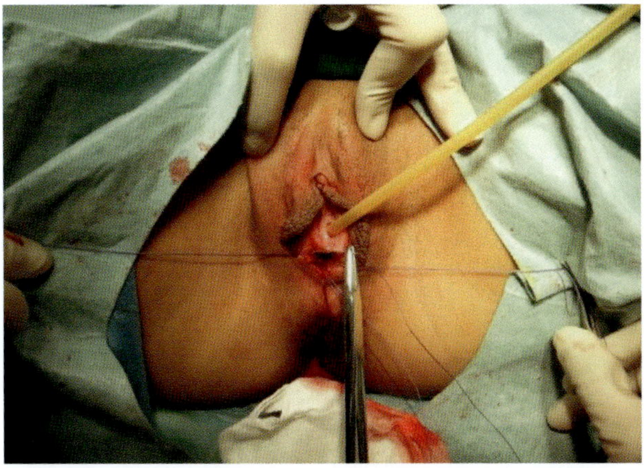

Fig. 4.53 The peritoneal membrane is stitched to the vaginal mucosa at the corresponding positions at the vaginal vestibule

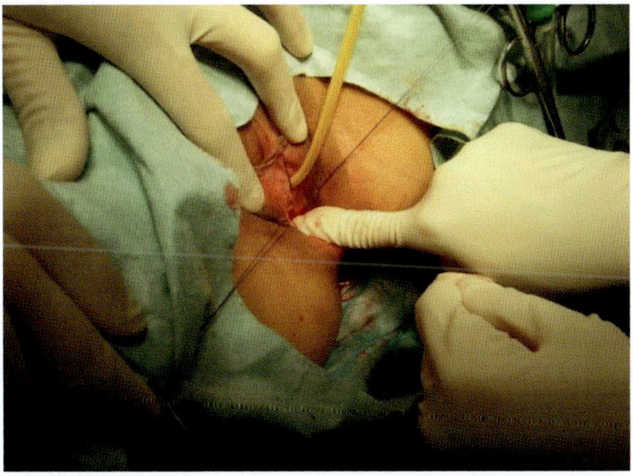

Fig. 4.54 All sutures are tied to approximate the peritoneal membrane and the mucosal membrane of the vaginal vestibule

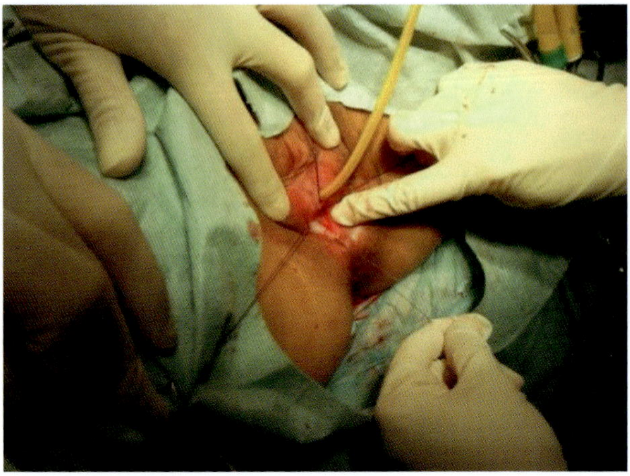

Fig. 4.55 Sutures are seen at respectively 12, 3, 6, and 9 o'clock positions

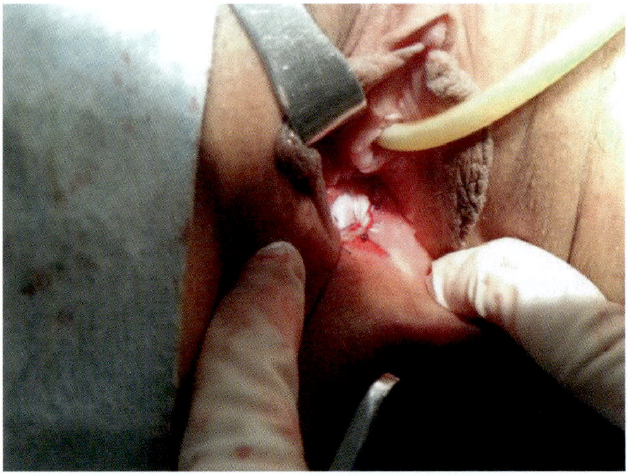

Fig. 4.56 The suturing of peritoneal membrane with the vaginal mucosa is completed and adequate hemostasis is observed

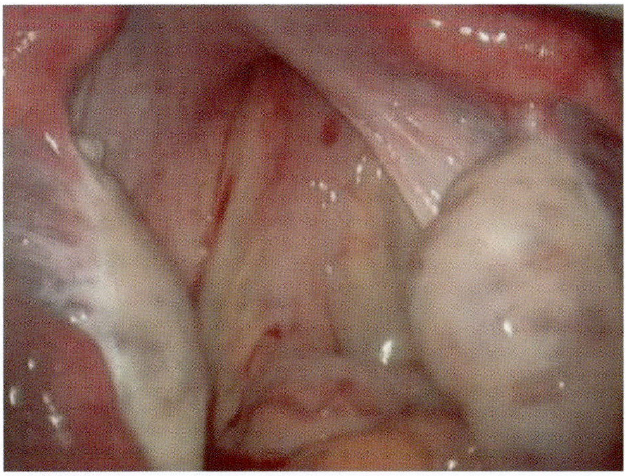

Fig. 4.57 The peritoneum of the pouch of Douglas has been pulled down and now it is covering the vaginal tunnel

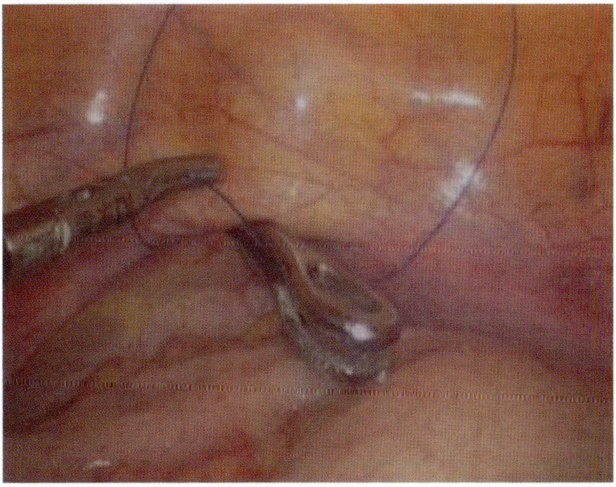

Fig. 4.58 A nonabsorbable Prolene 1/0 suture is inserted into the pelvis to close the pelvic floor peritoneum

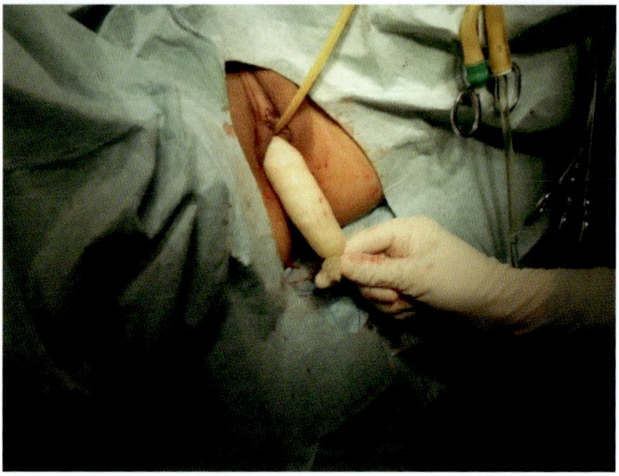

Fig. 4.59 A homemade vaginal mold is inserted into the new vagina

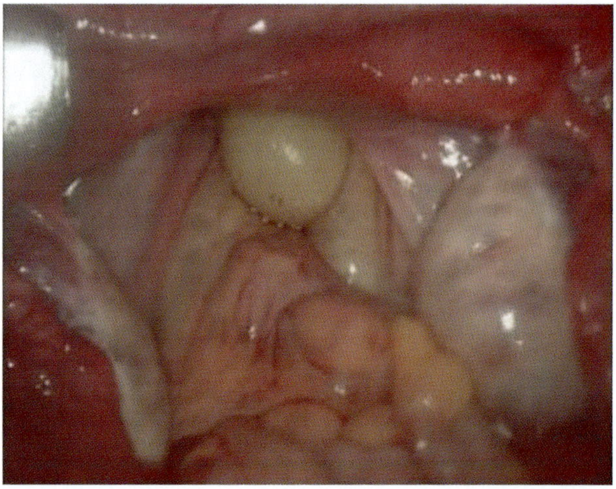

Fig. 4.60 The tip of the vaginal mold is positioned up to the level of fibrous cords in the pelvis

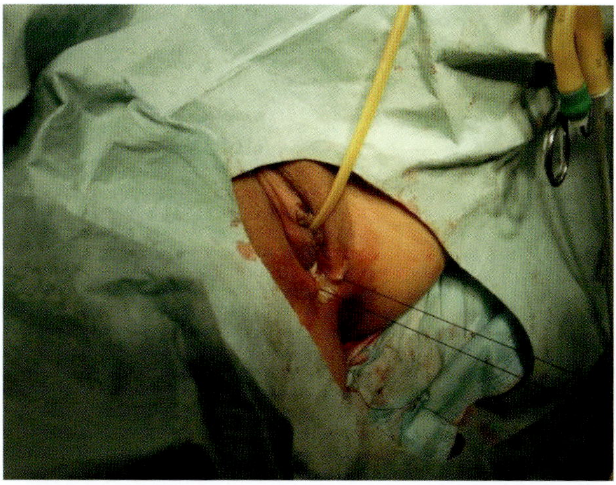

Fig. 4.61 The labia minora are sutured and closed to keep the vaginal mold in the vagina

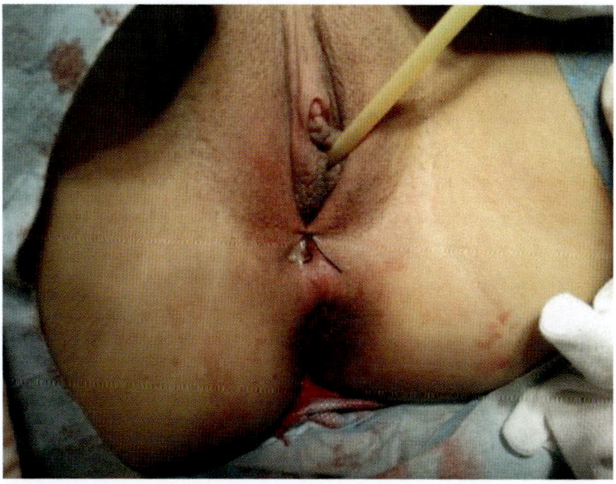

Fig. 4.62 A suture knot is tied to close the vaginal opening to prevent the vaginal mold from falling out of the vagina

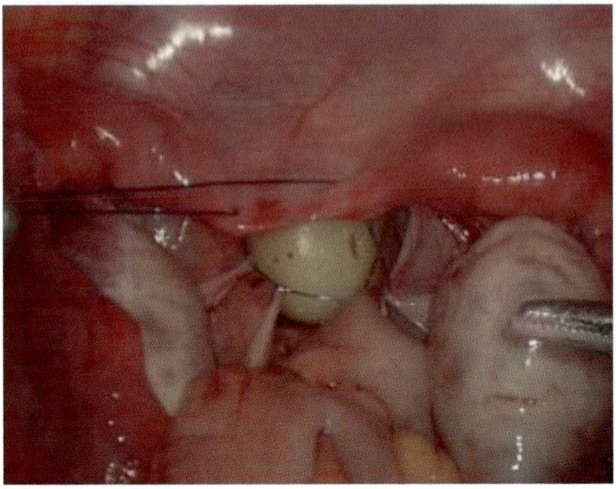

Fig. 4.63 A nonabsorbable Prolene suture is used to close the peritoneum of the pelvic floor with seven stitches purse-string suture method (practically, the seven stitches purse-string suture method involves the following: (*1*) the first stitch starts inserting the needle at 1 cm to the right of the center of the fibrous cords at the bottom level of the bladder; (*2*) the second stitch picks the side wall peritoneum below the right ovary; (*3*) the third stitch takes the peritoneum on the right side of the rectum; (*4*) the fourth stitch is at rectal wall about the level of the bottom of the bladder, the suture should penetrate only the serous muscular layer of the rectum; (*5*) the fifth stitch takes the peritoneum on the left of the rectum; (*6*) the sixth stitch at the peritoneal wall below the left ovary; (*7*) the final seventh stitch is at 1 cm to the left of the center of the fibrous cords at the bottom of the bladder

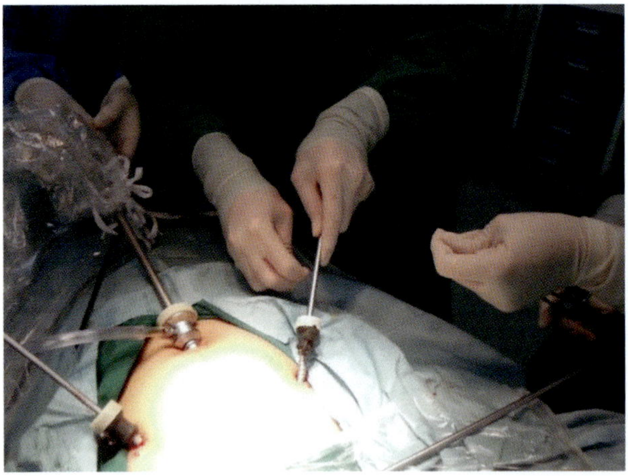

Fig. 4.64 The two ends of the above suture are delivered outside the abdomen via the cannula at the left lower cannula. An extracorporeal knot is tied and pushed down into the abdomen to form a taut purse-string suture to close the pelvic floor

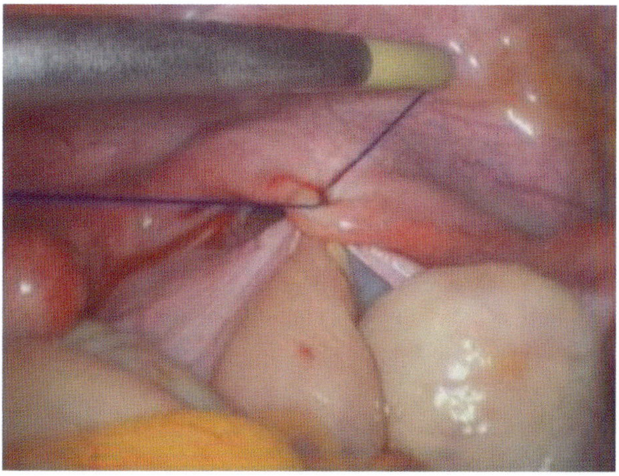

Fig. 4.65 The above suturing knot is secured by another intracorporeal counter knot

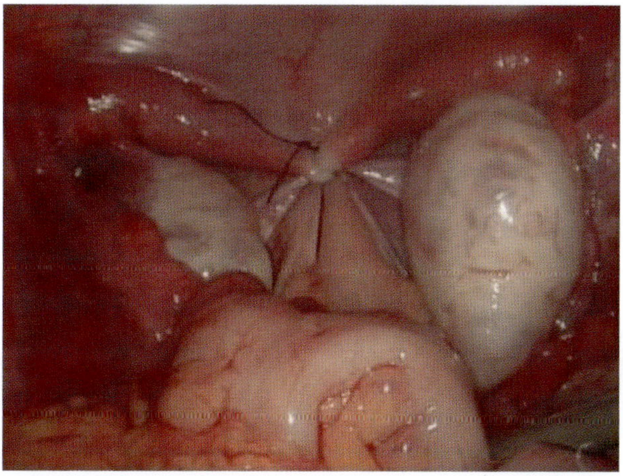

Fig. 4.66 Reformation of the pelvic floor, a new peritoneal top of the vagina. The surgery is completed

Key Points of Surgical Techniques

1. Before making the vaginal tunnel, sufficient water should be injected to form a large water cushion. The water cushion helps to separate the pelvic peritoneum around the internal vaginal opening. This will also reduce bleeding and avoid rectal injury during the creation of the vaginal tunnel (Figs. 4.23, 4.24, 4.25, 4.26, 4.27, and 4.28)
2. Vaginal dilators: Vaginal dilators are used to push up the pelvic peritoneum for the incision and progressively expand the tunnel and the peritoneal incision. This is the key technique of the surgery. This will result in less injury and bleeding with a new smooth vaginal tunnel

4.1.4.6 Postoperative Management

1. Appropriate postoperative antibiotic treatment.
2. Antiseptic solution (0.1 % iodophor) washing and preparation of the vulva and perineum twice a day after the operation.
3. The urinary catheter can be removed on day 2–3 after operation.
4. From the postoperative day 10, the vaginal mold can be removed. A urinary catheter is inserted into the vagina for washing it with 0.1 % iodophor daily for 3 days. Afterward, the patient should learn how to expand the vagina with a vaginal dilator once a day, 10 min each time. With the "Luo Hu style" vaginal dilators, a small-sized dilator is first used, followed by changing it to a medium-sized or a large-sized dilator according to the tightness of the vagina over a few days (Figs. 4.68, 4.69, 4.70, and 4.71). One to two months after operation, sexual activity can begin. The vaginal mold or dilator will not be required for those with regular sex.

4.1.4.7 Recovery Stages After Laparoscopic Peritoneal-Assisted Vaginoplasty

In practice, we observed that after peritoneal vaginoplasty, there are different time intervals presenting in different recovery stages. According to different appearances and characteristics of the new vagina, there are four recovery stages which can be managed accordingly. Appropriate postoperative management is very important to the future success and functionality of the new vagina. The recovery stages are described as follows:

Stage of Creation of the Vagina: 10–15 Days After Surgery

Characteristics
When the vaginal mold is removed, a new vagina has now formed. The vaginal peritoneum has now adhered to the surrounding tissues with the pelvic floor closed. During this period, the vagina is loose and deep, up to 12–15 cm.

Management
Daily vaginal wash is with 0.1 % iodophor. Each time, the vagina is examined by inserting the index finger into the vagina to feel and assess the vaginal condition inside. In the meantime, small-sized vaginal dilators can be used to expand the vagina.

Stage of Scar Contracture: 15–30 Days After Surgery

Characteristics
A large amount of connective tissues will form around the vagina, which become narrower, lighter, and hardened. Pathological examination of the vagina will show fibrous connective tissue and inflammatory cells, but no epithelial cells. The depth of the vagina is now about 7–9 cm.

Management
Every day, a lubricated and gloved index finger is inserted into the vagina to expand it. At the beginning, the vagina may feel very tight and can accommodate only one finger. The anastomotic opening is narrow, allowing only one finger for an in and out expansion. After a few days, there is a gradual relaxation of the vagina. A small-sized vaginal dilator can then be used to replace the digital expansion. Patients should be taught to expand the vaginas by themselves. Every day, a vaginal dilator can be used to expand the vagina 1–2 times, 10 min each time (Figs. 4.68, 4.69, 4.70, and 4.71).

Each time after performing the vaginal expansion, there may be some vaginal bleeding which is self-limiting. The bleeding will stop on its own. After vaginal expansion, the vagina should be scrubbed with povidone-iodine cotton stick to prevent infection. This stage is the most important stage for vaginal expansion, usually under the guidance of a doctor. The patient should remain hospitalized for this period of time. It is therefore inappropriate to discharge her from hospital too early. At the same time, this patient should be provided with sexual and psychological counseling. If this stage is not properly handled, the depth of the vagina and the future sex life can be affected.

Stage of Relaxing and Softening: 30 Days and 3 Months After Surgery

Characteristics
The connective tissues around the vagina begin to be resorbed and become softened. The vagina is now soft and flexible and gradually deeper and wider. The depth of the vagina at this stage is about 8–12 cm.

Management
At this stage, the patient is generally discharged home and has returned to normal work and life. She can use a small- or a medium-sized vaginal dilator to expand the vagina, once every day, with a 10 min duration. Bleeding is gradually reduced to scanty and even nothing. Generally after 2 months, majority of patients can have sex life. If so, it may replace the use of vaginal dilators with even better effect.

Stage of Vaginal Maturity: 3 Months After Surgery

Characteristics
The vagina becomes increasingly soften and elastic with some vaginal folds appearing. There are also some milky whitish vaginal discharges covering the pink vaginal mucous membrane (Fig. 4.72). Pathological examination of the vaginal mucosa showed stratified squamous epithelium. The laparoscopic wounds will now become hardly visible (Fig. 4.73).

Management
From this time onward, the vagina will no longer collapse or close. No special treatment is required for marriage and sexual intercourse. If without sex life, a vaginal dilator may be used one to two times a week or patient may expand the vagina with her own index and middle fingers during bath.

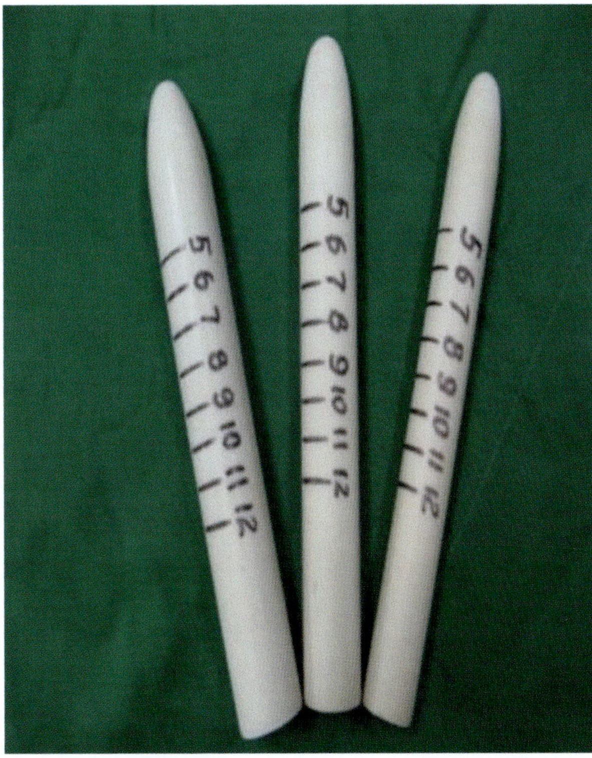

Fig. 4.67 "Luo Hu style" vaginal dilators with scale marking (for patient use); specifications: length 20 cm; diameter: small 2.2 cm, medium 2.5 cm, large 2.8 cm

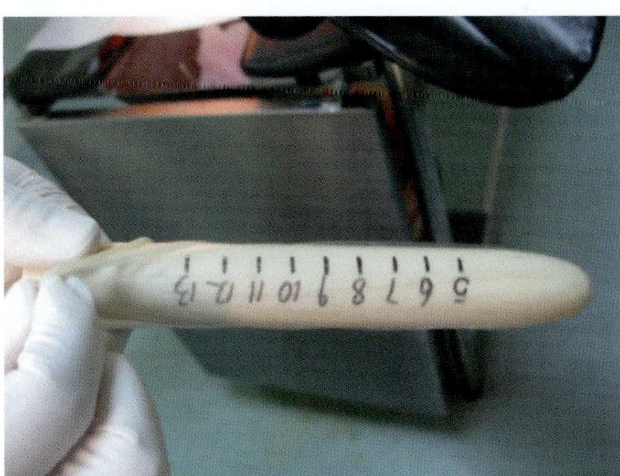

Fig. 4.68 A vaginal dilator is put into a condom and lubricant is smeared onto the head of the dilator

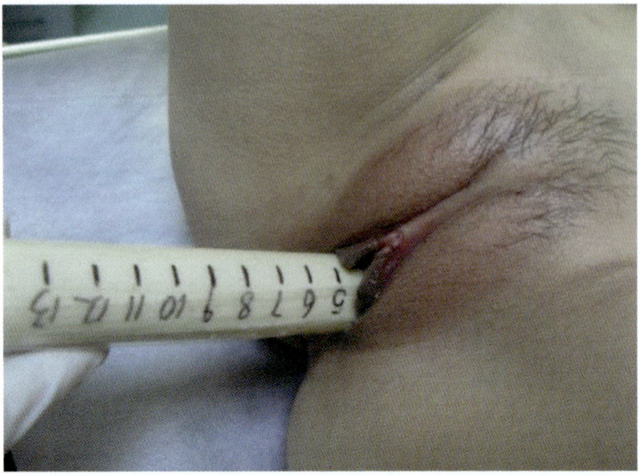

Fig. 4.69 The vaginal dilator is now gradually put into the vagina

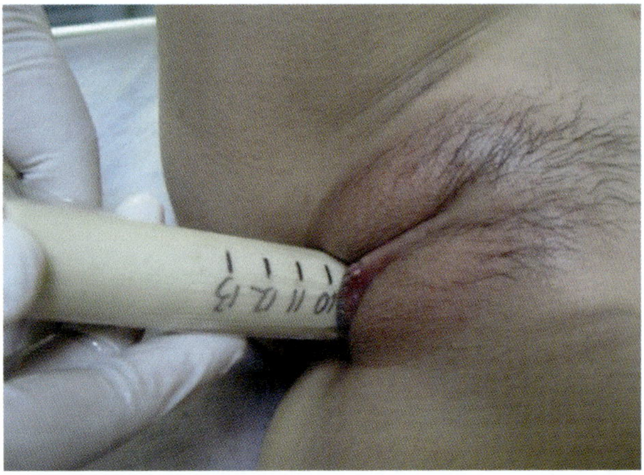

Fig. 4.70 The dilator is pushed slightly harder till reaching the top end of the vagina. Then in and out movements are performed repeatedly, for 5–10 min duration

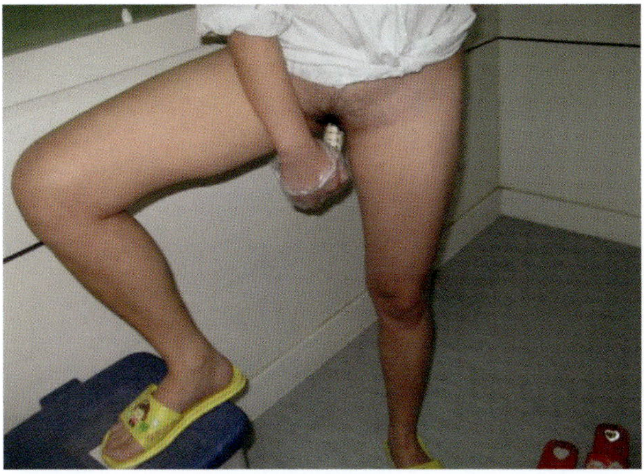

Fig. 4.71 Patient can easily perform the vaginal expansion herself by partly standing up on one leg, with another leg stepping on a small stool as shown

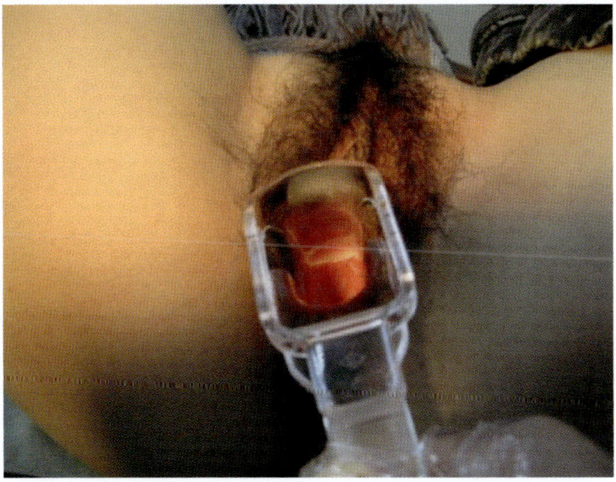

Fig. 4.72 Six months after surgery, the vagina becomes elastic and folds appear. The vagina shows pink vaginal mucous membrane and some milky white discharge

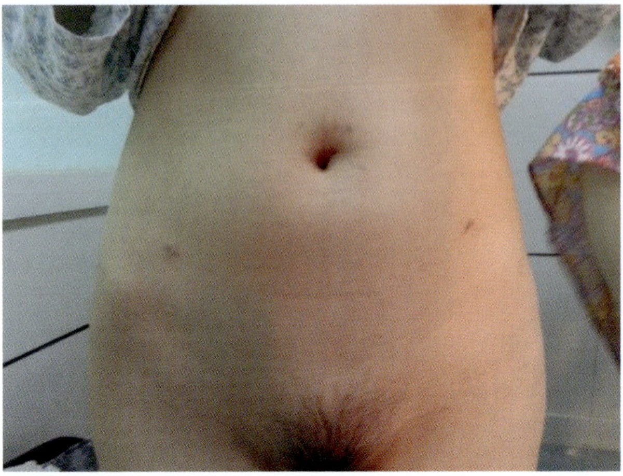

Fig. 4.73 The laparoscopic wound scars will gradually heal well and become hardly visible after a few months

4.1.5 *Transvaginal Peritoneal Vaginoplasty*

Hang Mei Jin

4.1.5.1 The Structure and Functions of the Peritoneum

Peritoneum is a serous membrane, consisting of the mesothelium lining the peritoneal cavity and the connective tissues underneath. It covers the inner wall of the abdomen and pelvis and the surfaces of the internal organs. It is a thin, transparent, smooth, and shiny layer of tissue. According to its areas of coverage, it can be divided into parietal peritoneum and the visceral peritoneum. The parietal peritoneum covers the abdominal wall, the pelvic wall, and underneath the diaphragm; the visceral peritoneum wraps around the internal organs and forms the serosal layers of all internal organs. They are connected in continuation as a peritoneal sac. In male, the peritoneal sac is completely closed, but in female, the peritoneal sac opening of the fallopian tubes is connected outside via the uterine and vaginal cavities. The irregular spaces between the visceral peritoneal layers and parietal peritoneal layers are called the peritoneal cavity. In addition to supporting and fixing the internal organs, the peritoneum also has the function of secretion and absorption. Under normal circumstances, peritoneum secretes a small amount of serous fluid to lubricate the surface of the organs, hence reducing friction of their movements. Peritoneal surface area is huge, especially the parietal peritoneum which covers the abdominal wall and pelvic floor, but their attachments to these walls are loose and can be easily separated.

As the peritoneal cavity has a very large surface area, it has a strong absorptive capacity. In pathological cases, an increase in peritoneal exudation from these surfaces may form ascites. Peritoneum also defends the body from harms, with some peritoneal cells having phagocytic function, and also when the abdominal organs have infection and are infectious, peritoneal tissues especially the omentum can quickly move to the infectious lesions, to adhere to them, and to engulf and localize the infection from spreading.

Peritoneum is rich in nerve receptors. The spinal nerves that dominate the parietal peritoneum also dominate the corresponding segments of the skin and body; touching, temperature, or chemical stimulation in the parietal peritoneum can induce pain in conscious patients. When the parietal peritoneum is irritated, there are reflex contractions in the abdominal muscle, resulting in a rigid abdominal wall phenomenon, i.e., guarding tenderness. The nerve that dominates the visceral peritoneum comes from the autonomic nervous system that dominates the internal organs and the visceral afferent nerves. They have different sensitivity to different stimuli.

The peritoneum also has a strong ability to repair and heal. Peritoneal mesothelial cells can be transformed into fiber cells. At different levels, the merger of the fibroblasts of peritoneal mesothelial origin is the basis of the strong peritoneal regeneration ability. Therefore, for gastrointestinal surgeries, a good serosal suture can allow a smooth contact surface and a faster healing and lesser adhesion. If surgery is rough, the peritoneum may be injured resulting in postoperative peritoneal adhesion.

Since the peritoneal membrane has the above special features, it provides a theoretic and practical basis for the peritoneal membrane to form a new vaginal wall. At present, there are basically four approaches:

1. By laparoscopic approach, the pelvic peritoneum is pushed down and fixed to the vaginal opening at the vaginal vestibule (under laparoscopy, a surgical procedure using a peritoneum pusher rod); the upper end of the new vagina is then sutured and closed by laparoscopic suturing.
2. By a combination of vaginal and laparoscopic approach, a vaginal tunnel between the bladder and rectum is created. The pelvic peritoneum is pulled down to the vagina and fixed to the vaginal mucosa at the vaginal vestibule. The upper end of the new vagina is then closed by laparoscopic suturing. This is the Luo Hu procedure as described in the last section.
3. By the vaginal approach, the pelvic peritoneum is pulled through the space between the bladder and rectum and fixed to the vaginal opening at the vaginal vestibule. The upper end of the new vagina is then closed by laparoscopic suturing.
4. By only the vaginal approach, a vaginal tunnel is created and the pelvic peritoneum is pulled down through the space between the bladder and rectum and fixed to the vaginal opening at the vaginal vestibule. The upper end of the new vagina is also closed by vaginal suturing. The last approach will be highlighted as follows the transvaginal peritoneal vaginoplasty.

4.1.5.2 Preoperative Assessment of Transvaginal Peritoneal Vaginoplasty

In 1933, Ksido pioneered peritoneal vaginoplasty. Through continuous improvement, this approach is considered better than the other operations; besides, it is not a complicated procedure. The key point is that when the new vaginal tunnel is created, the patient's own pelvic peritoneum is used to cover the vaginal tunnel to complete vaginoplasty. The success of this operation is the selection of patients. The surgical technique is now better developed, leading to significant improvement to free the pelvic peritoneum, to push it down as well as to close the vaginal vault.

If the pelvic peritoneum is more slack over a large area, it is then feasible to perform a relatively simple transvaginal peritoneal vaginoplasty. The key surgical techniques of this operation are that the freeing, pulling down of pelvic peritoneum, as well as the closure of the vaginal vault are completed within the newly created vagina. It is a minimally invasive procedure and leaves no abdominal surgical scar.

After years of practices, Dr. Sun Jin and his colleagues from the department of Obstetrics and Gynecology, Zhejiang University Hospital, had reached a satisfactory sexual function of 82.4 % after 20 years of follow-up. In order to guarantee a successful operation and satisfactory postoperative result, they proposed that before the operation, patients should be assessed on the size of the area and the degree of laxity of the pelvic peritoneum. They classified three types of pelvic peritoneum for this procedure.

1. During rectal examination, a gloved index finger should pass deep into the rectum till reaching the pelvic peritoneum. At the junction of the primordial uteri on both sides, there is generally a palpable cordlike peritoneal folding band. If that can be

reached by the finger, then with the tip of the index finger it should be hooked and pulled toward the anus (Fig. 4.74). If it can be pulled down for more than 2 cm, then it is a type I pelvic peritoneum, suggesting that pelvic peritoneum is more slack and can be freed for a larger area so that the surgery can be more easily performed and be successful. If the cordlike peritoneal folding band can be reached and pulled down with the hooked index fingertip but only slightly for less than 2 cm, it is a type II pelvic peritoneum, suggesting that the pelvic peritoneum is tight and can be freed for only a smaller area. Even the surgery can be successful, there may be some difficulties to perform. An experienced surgeon is required to perform this procedure to achieve a successful outcome. In some patients, suturing at the top end of the new vaginal tunnel may be more difficult; it might have to be done via the abdomen and perhaps under the laparoscope to avoid ending with a short vagina. If the index finger deep at the pelvic floor yet it cannot touch the cordlike peritoneal folding band, this is a pelvic peritoneum type III. For this group of patients, the pelvic peritoneum is either too tight or too high that only little area can be freed to allow the surgery to be completed successfully. If the surgeon does not have great experience in this surgical approach, it should be abandoned. He/She should consider other surgical approaches such as the sigmoid colon vaginoplasty or the biological patches (acellular dermal matrix) vaginoplasty.

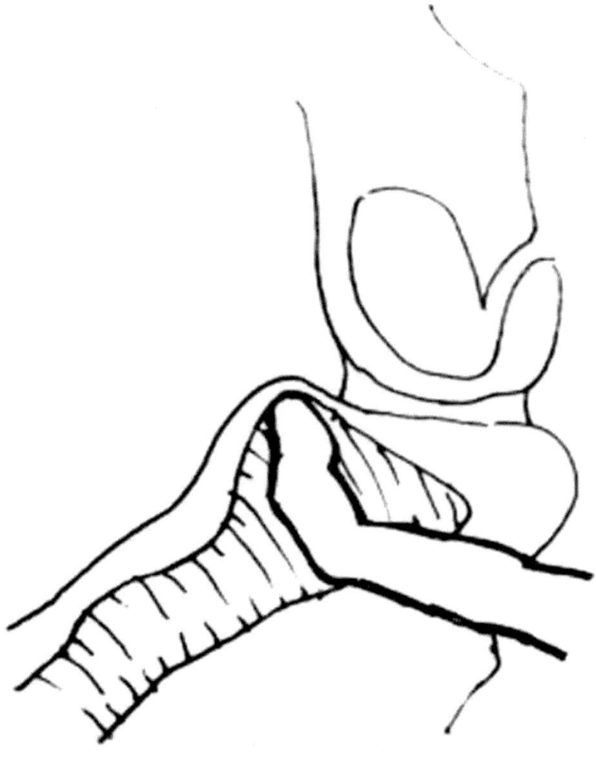

Fig. 4.74 A method to assess the laxity of the pelvic peritoneum

4.1.5.3 Surgical Procedures, Techniques, and Postoperative Management

Surgical Procedures

All surgical procedures are performed vaginally.

(a) With the patient in a lithotomy position, a curved incision of about 4 cm is made at the depressed center of the vaginal vestibule (Figs. 4.75 and 4.76). The mucosa and underlying connective tissue at the vestibule are incised by using a pair of forceps to lift the upper vestibular mucosa; a sharp cut will open the mucosal membrane and its connective tissues underneath. An index finger is then inserted into the incised wound and pushed into the space of loose tissues between the bladder and the rectum. If the surgical plane is correct, the intervening tissues are loose and can be easily separated.

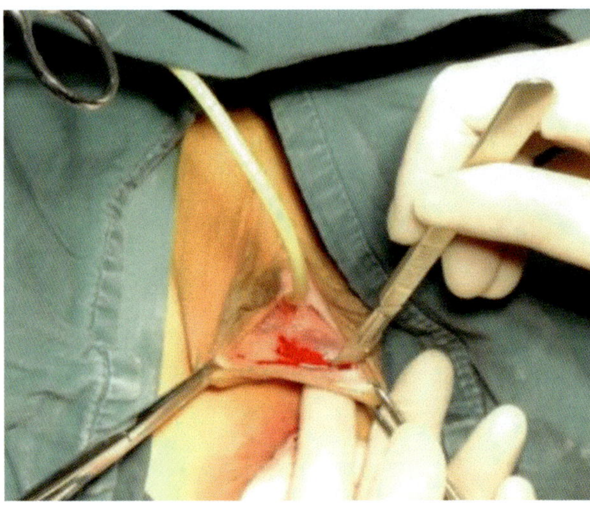

Fig. 4.75 A curved incision is made at the vaginal vestibule

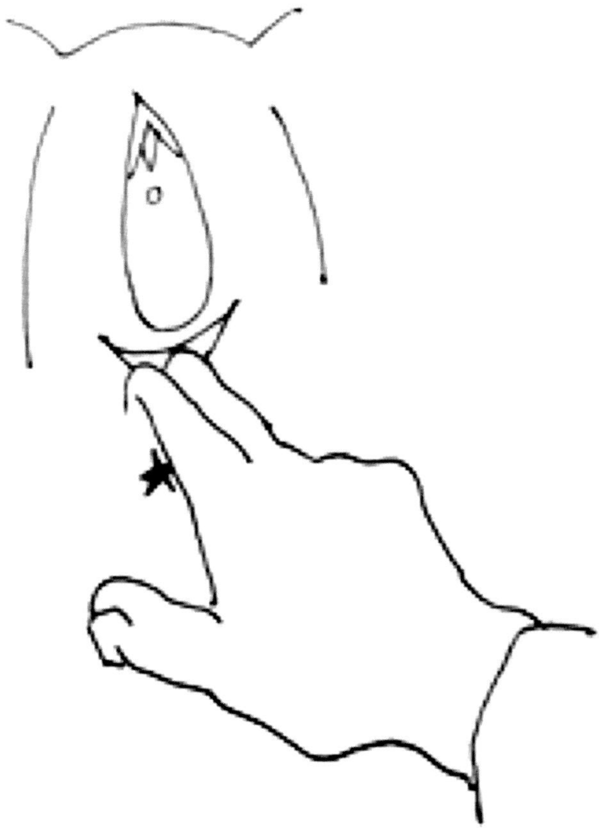

Fig. 4.76 The index and middle fingers are inserted and pushed forward to open the loose tissues between the bladder and rectum

(b) The creation of a vaginal tunnel: When making a vaginal tunnel, it is important to find the appropriate anatomical plane. The index fingers of both hands are inserted and pushed forward in a horizontal and slightly upward direction, bluntly freeing the loose tissues in the space among the urethra, the bladder in front, and the rectum behind for up to 3–4 cm. The two fingers are then moving bluntly to the left and right, respectively, and advancing forward to free the loose tissues until reaching the pelvic peritoneum. The vaginal tunnel should be wide enough to accommodate three fingers across (Figs. 4.77 and 4.78). The vaginal tunnel should be packed with dry gauze which can provide pressure to stop any bleeding.
(c) The bulbospongiosus on both sides of the incision at the vaginal vestibule are lifted up with tissue forceps; they are partially cut to allow adequate lateral extension of the vaginal tunnel opening. The cut edges of bulbospongiosus are sutured to stop bleeding.
(d) The dry gauze which has been inserted into the vaginal tunnel can now be removed, and two vaginal retractors of 12 cm long are used to retract the bladder in front and the rectum behind, to expose the top end of the vaginal tunnel. A long tissue scissors can now shear the loose tissues at the top end of the tunnel, until the pelvic peritoneum is visible like an amniotic sac bulging slightly into the tunnel. A long curved vascular forceps can be used to clamp and release the peritoneum to make a visible forceps mark on the membrane; the marking will confirm it as the pelvic peritoneum.

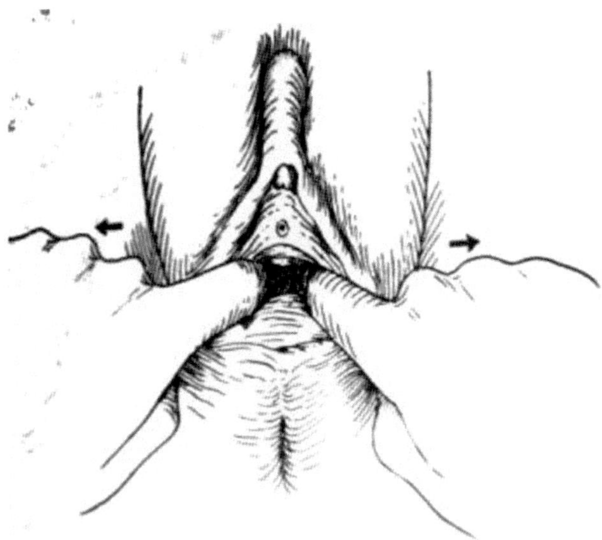

Fig. 4.77 A vaginal tunnel is being made by two fingers separating the loose tissues between the bladder and rectum

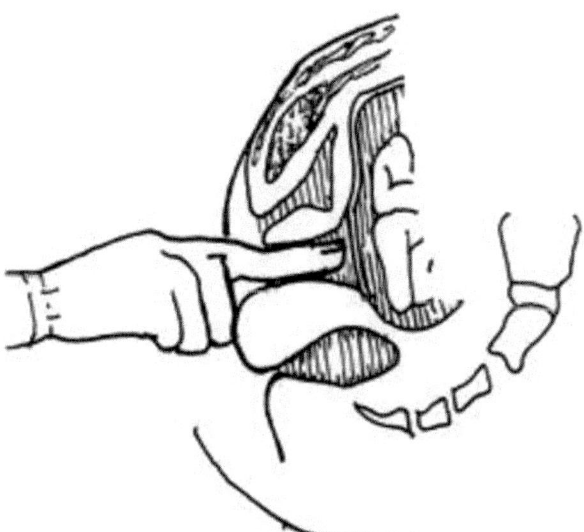

Fig. 4.78 Separation of loose tissues in the gap between bladder and rectum till reaching the pelvic peritoneum

(e) A pair of long tissue scissors is used to cut open the pelvic peritoneum (Fig. 4.79) which has a very smooth surface, then a small amount of peritoneal fluid can be seen flowing out. After confirming this is the peritoneum, the incision is expanded by putting a left index finger deep into the peritoneal incision. Under the guidance of the index finger, the bladder is pushed up, the cordlike muscle tissue from the reverse-folding peritoneal belt is freed, cut, and ligated (for some patients, it is a primordial uterus). Only when the cordlike muscle tissue of the reverse-folding peritoneal belt has been cut off, the pelvic peritoneum can be freed from the pelvic floor more easily.

While freeing the pelvic peritoneum, the opening of the peritoneum is expanded, so that its size matches the size of the vaginal vestibule incision. Only with sufficiently freed pelvic peritoneum, it can prevent vaginal stenosis shortly after the operation.

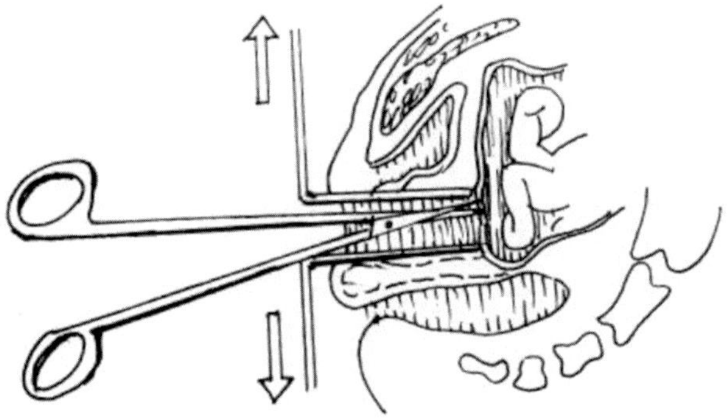

Fig. 4.79 When the pelvic peritoneum is exposed via the vaginal tunnel, it is cut opened by a long tissue scissors

6. The freed pelvic peritoneum is pulled down through the vaginal tunnel to the corresponding positions at the vaginal opening at the vestibule. Using 3/0 absorbable sutures, the edges of the peritoneal membrane and the vaginal mucosa are sutured together with interrupted stitches, to form a new vaginal opening (Figs. 4.80 and 4.81). Examination will now show a vagina of about 10 cm long and accommodate two fingers loosely. The vaginal surface lining is smooth as it is the pelvic peritoneum (Fig. 4.82).

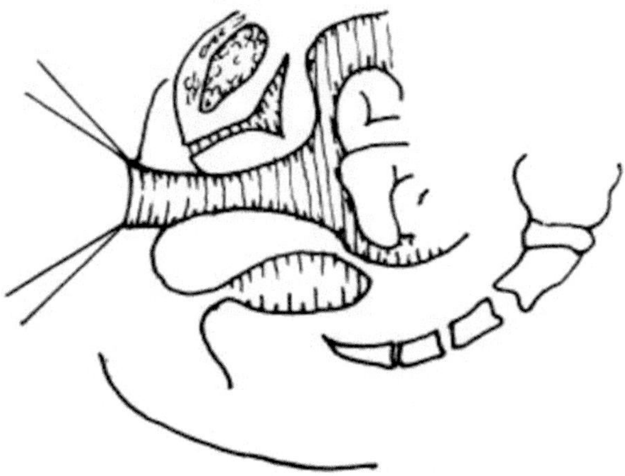

Fig. 4.80 The pelvic peritoneum was pulled down and sutured to the vaginal mucosa so as to cover the whole vaginal tunnel

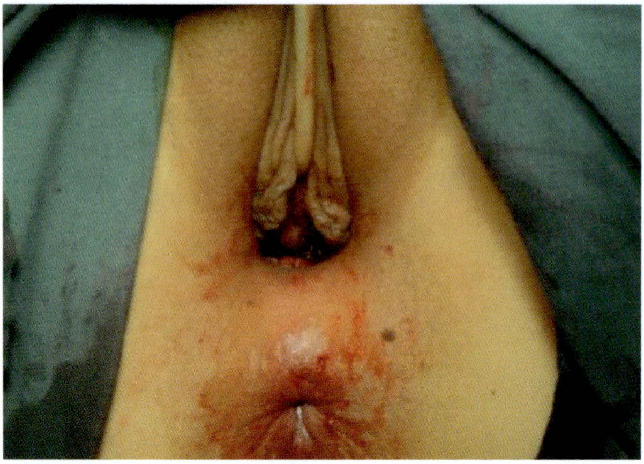

Fig. 4.81 The creation of a new vaginal opening

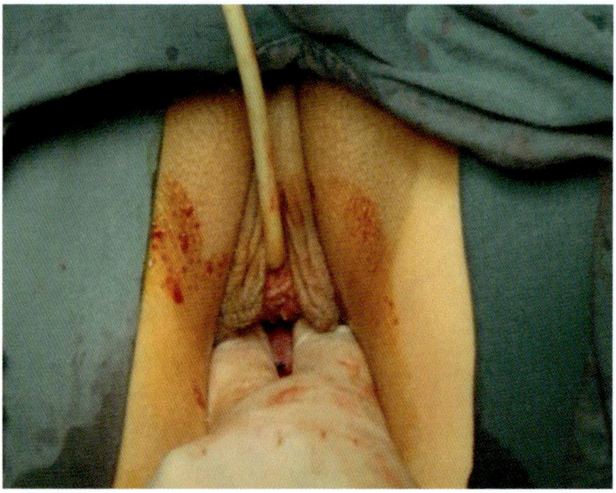

Fig. 4.82 Examination showed a vagina of 10 cm long, accommodating two fingers easily, with smooth pelvic peritoneum covering it

7. Two vaginal retractors of 12 cm long are inserted into the newly formed vaginal tunnel to enlarge the tunnel and use of a long needle holder with 2/0 absorbable suture to suture the top of the peritoneum at a point about 10 cm from the vaginal opening. Half purse-string sutures are put into the two corners of the pelvic peritoneal opening to close the peritoneum at the vaginal vault. Then another 2/0 absorbable suture is used as a continuous suture to reinforce the strength of the new vaginal vault (Fig. 4.83).

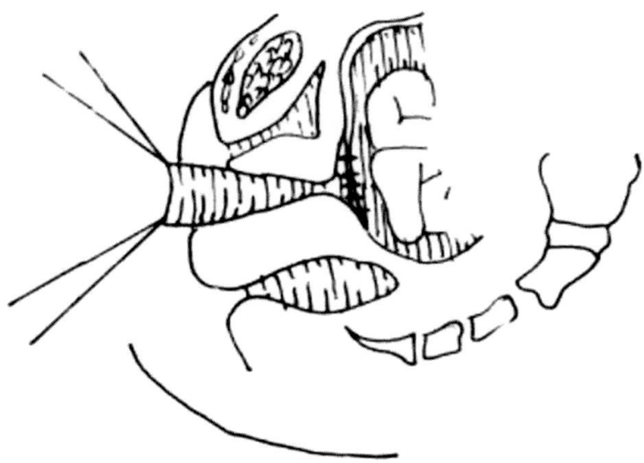

Fig. 4.83 The pelvic peritoneum at 10 cm depth is closed by operating through the vagina to form a new vaginal vault

8. A Foley catheter is inserted into the bladder to examine the urine for any urethral and bladder injury. Digital examination of the rectum is also performed to ensure no suture has penetrated through the rectum. When any injury to these organs is excluded, a soft homemade vaginal mold can be put into the new vagina in order to distend it and to stop bleeding by pressure. The vaginal mold can be created and used as shown in Figs. 4.84, 4.85, and 4.86.
9. A sterile gauze pad is now placed over the vulva, and a T-band supporter is worn to prevent the soft vaginal mold from slipping out. The operation is now complete.

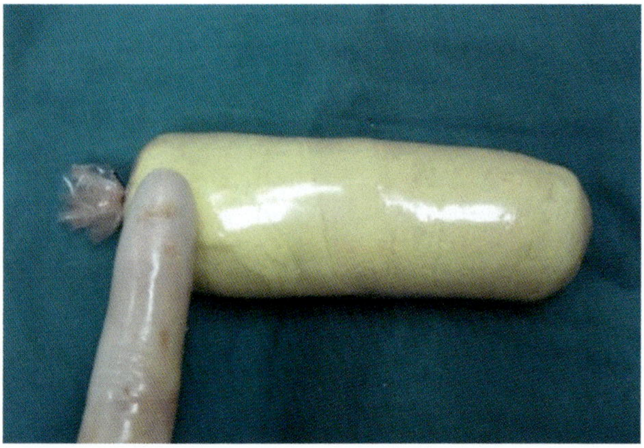

Fig. 4.84 A soft homemade vaginal mold is created by packing rolled up povidone-iodine gauzes into a condom

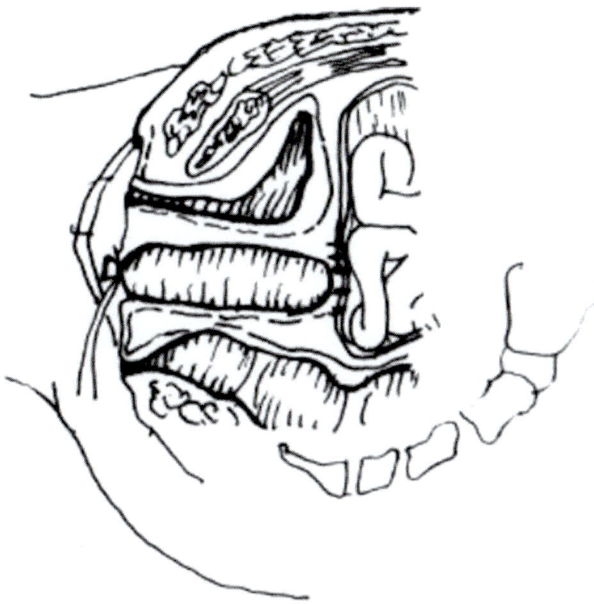

Fig. 4.85 A soft vaginal mold is put into the new vagina

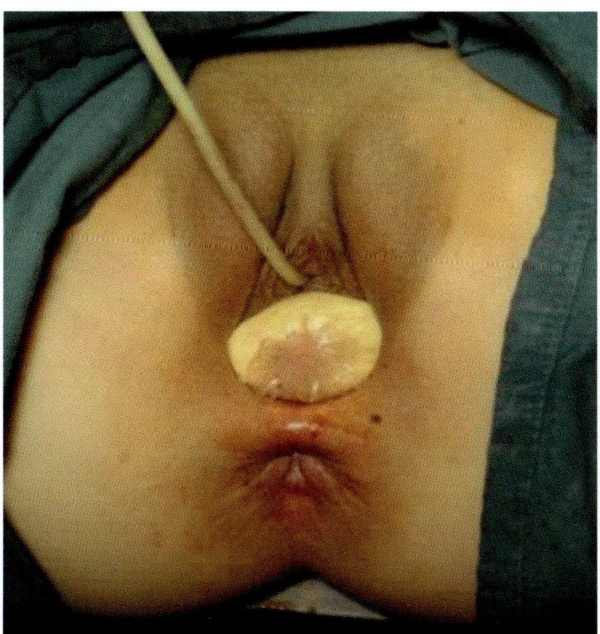

Fig. 4.86 A soft vaginal mold is inserted in the new vagina

4.1.5.4 Postoperative Management

Routine prophylactic antibiotic is used in vulvovaginal surgery to prevent infection. Fluid diet is allowed on day 1 after surgery; then it can be changed to soft diet when flatus has passed. On 3–5 days after operation, the Foley catheter can be removed. On the seventh day, the vaginal mold or soft plug is removed from the vagina. The vulva and vagina are cleansed with 5 % povidone-iodine daily. The vaginal mold is used continuously to expand the new vagina for no less than 3 months, even after discharged home from the hospital. The patient will be instructed to change the mold herself, and for the unmarried, to do it until there is regular sex life.

The author also recommends the use of a hard mold (Fig. 4.87), measuring 4 cm in diameter and 10 cm in length. The mold is made of nontoxic polypropylene materials, very lightweight, and smooth. It has an empty cavity with a finger-sized hole at the end. It is slightly curved with a groove on the side facing the urethra, to avoid compression to the urethra leading to difficulty to pass urine (Fig. 4.87). The mold is light, smooth, and tilt as the reproductive tract; it has the advantages of easy cleansing, changing, and carrying.

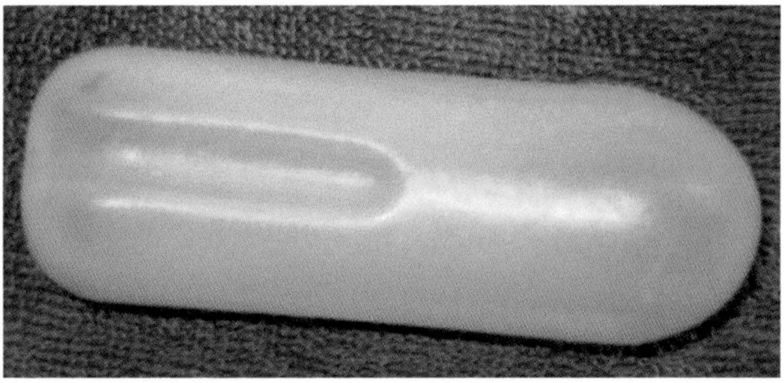

Fig. 4.87 A hard vaginal mold measuring 10 × 4 cm, with a groove surface facing the urethra when inserted in the vagina

4.1.5.5 Follow-Up

It is very important for patients to be followed up and reassessed at the hospital at 1, 3, and 6 months and 1 year. They are mainly for the assessment of the depth and width of the vagina, especially attention is paid to observe any granulation tissue at the top of the vagina and to give advice for the use of mold. For patients with sex life, the quality of sexual life, e.g., sexual desire, orgasm, vaginal length, vaginal wetness, and the sex satisfaction, is assessed. If necessary, psychological support and guidance of sex life are offered to these patients.

This is a simple transvaginal peritoneal vaginoplasty procedure which is minimally invasive and scarless. Its advantages are quick recovery and good cosmetic cover-up without surgical scars. From our study of 300 cases with a follow-up period of 5–20 years, the satisfaction on the quality of sex life is more than 80 %.

It is noteworthy that preoperative assessment to the types of pelvic peritoneum and its laxity is important to choose an appropriate surgical procedure. Besides, whether the surgeon is familiar with the procedure and can master the technique or not are the keys to success. It is important to classify the pelvic peritoneum into different types, where type I and type II pelvic peritoneum are loose over a wide area of the pelvic floor and are easy to pull down through the vaginal tunnel, enabling this approach to be successful. While type III has a high and tight pelvic peritoneum, resulting in a high failure rate with this approach, therefore the procedure should be changed to other more appropriate procedure. Preoperative bowel preparation is important because the surgery may damage the rectum in order to minimize bowel complications.

When making a vaginal tunnel, it is important to find the correct anatomical plane to avoid injury to the rectum and the bladder. Freeing the pelvic peritoneum sufficiently is the key to prevent stenosis or shortening of the new vagina after the operation. To prevent the postoperative vaginal stenosis, the use of a vaginal mold to expand the new vagina, and its wearing, should not be less than 3 months after discharged from hospital. Patients are advised to wear the mold till they get married or have regular sexual intercourses. To gain patients' cooperation, it is very important to provide postoperative assistance, counseling, and psychological supports to the patients or their parents to emphasize that the success of the operation depends on the persistent use of the vaginal mold. Postoperative follow-up is very important to help patients who may develop vaginal granulation in the vaginal vault, and hence affecting the healing of the new vagina. Granulation tissue should be promptly cut and removed. Follow-up after marriage is mainly for psychological support and guidance of sex life.

4.1.6 Laparoscopic Ileal Vaginoplasty

Li Bin and Huan-ying Wang

4.1.6.1 Total Laparoscopic Ileal Vaginoplasty

Surgical Procedures

1. Traditional abdominal and vulval disinfection, draping the surgical parts, and inserting an indwelling urinary catheter into the bladder are performed prior to the surgery.
2. CO_2 pneumoperitoneum is established to maintain the intra-abdominal pressure at 12–13 mmHg.
3. Depending on the distance between the umbilicus and the pubic symphysis and on whether there is any previous abdominal surgery, etc., one has to decide the position of the primary portal entry. Generally, the port is chosen at the center of the navel or at its upper/lower edge. If necessary, the midpoint of the line from the umbilicus to the xiphoid sternum can be chosen for the insertion of primary trocar and cannula.
4. A full examination of the abdominal and pelvic organs is performed including bilateral fallopian tubes, ovaries, kidneys, and ileum, as well as to find out if there is a primordial uterus (Fig. 4.88) or free kidney.

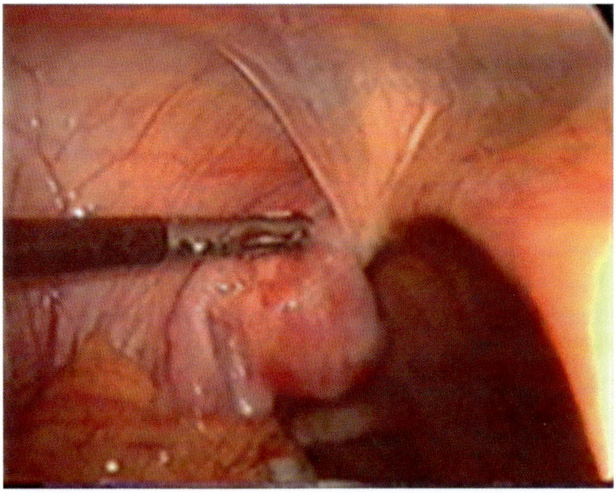

Fig. 4.88 Primordial uterus

5. After a full laparoscopic examination, insertion of operative instruments can be performed by puncturing and inserting the instruments one by one, under the supervision of laparoscope. Three other accessory portal positions are commonly at the lower left and right abdomen, on the left above the pubis. The trocars and cannulas used are with sizes 5.5 and 10 mm, respectively.
6. A segment of ileal loop located at about 50 cm from the ileocecal junction is chosen, freed, and to be transplanted; it will be 13–15 cm long supported by independent vessels. Ultrasonic knife is used to free the ileal mesentery, taking care to preserve the vascular arch so as to avoid ischemia and vascular necrosis (Fig. 4.89). If there is any bleeding, it can be stopped by ultrasonic knife, electric coagulation, or titanium clipping techniques (Fig. 4.90).

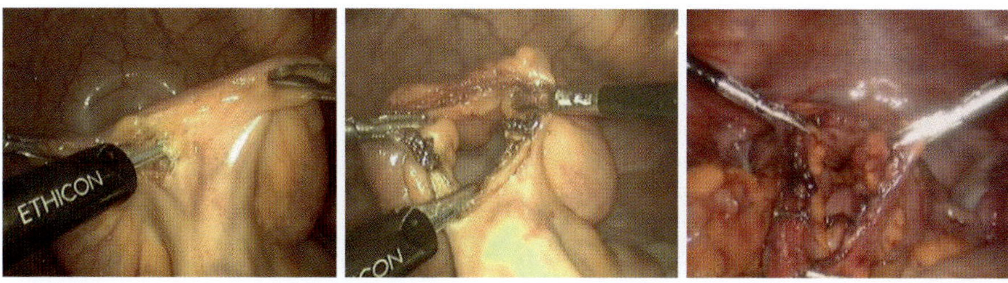

Fig. 4.89 Freeing a segment of ileum with ultrasonic scalpel

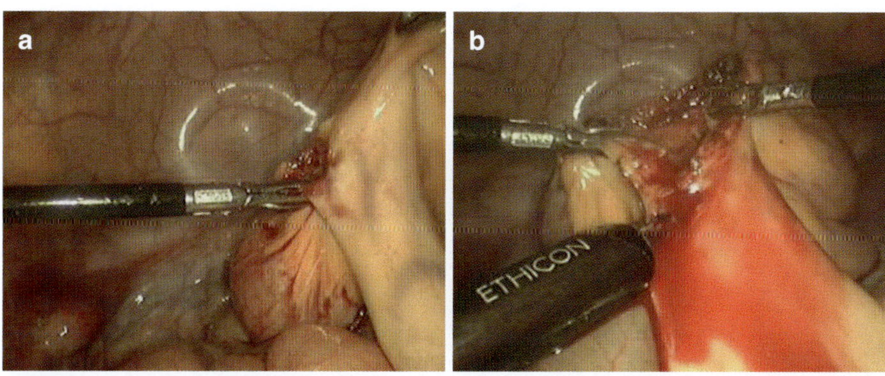

Fig. 4.90 Coagulation of bleeding points with (**a**) bipolar electric coagulation or (**b**) ultrasonic scalpel

7. Cutting and transplanting the ileal loop, suturing the two open ends of ileum:

   An endocutter is used to cut off an ileal loop for the ileal vaginoplasty (Fig. 4.91a–d) and another endocutter to achieve functional anastomosis of the two open ends of the remaining ileum (Fig. 4.92); or under laparoscope, the two ends of the ileum are sutured together by the traditional laparoscopic bowel anastomosis technique. The surgical procedures are shown as in Fig. 4.93 and are briefly described as follows (Fig. 4.93). Using a No. 1 Vicryl thread, the seromuscular layers of the two open ends in the ileum are sutured together. Through the trocar, the ileum is lifted up in the abdominal cavity (Fig. 4.93a). An ultrasonic scalpel is used to excise the two closed ends of the ileum to open the ends (Fig. 4.93c). The two ends of the ilea are closed together with full-thickness interrupted sutures (Fig. 4.93d, e). Similarly, the seromuscular layers of both ilea are sutured by interrupted stitches (Fig. 4.93b, f). No. 1 Vicryl thread is used to close the ileal mesentery (Fig. 4.94). The location and appearance of anastomosis are checked whether it meets anatomical requirements. If there is any primordial uterus, it can be excised and removed with the ultrasonic scalpel.

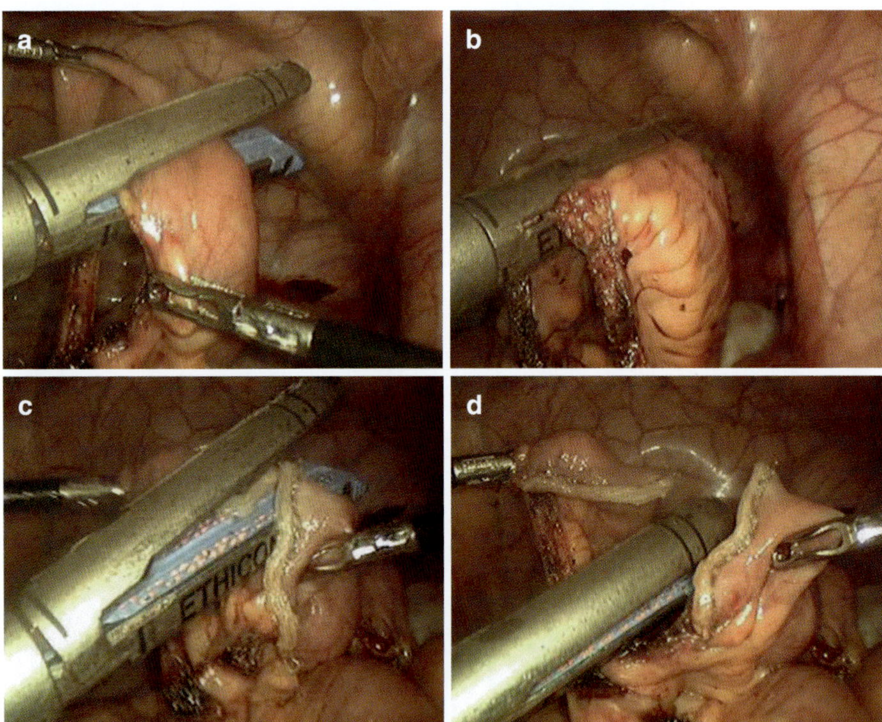

Fig. 4.91 Endocutter is used to cut and separate a segment of the ileum for the ileal vaginoplasty. (**a**) A segment of the ileum is placed between the blades of the endocutter. (**b**) The endocutter is ready to cut the ileum. (**c**, **d**) The ileum is completely cut apart and separated

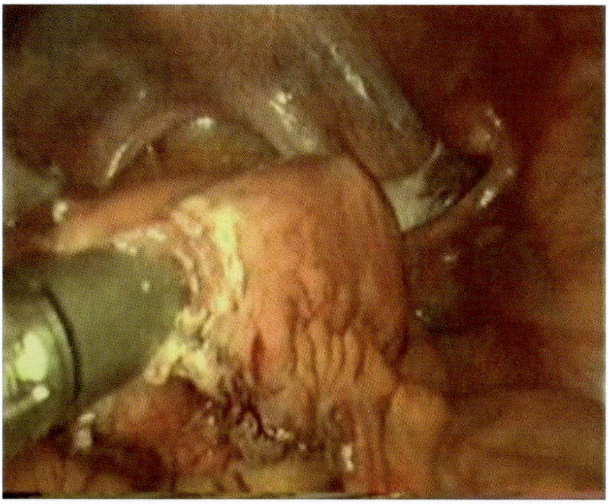

Fig. 4.92 An endocutter is used laparoscopically to achieve a functional anastomosis of the two ends of the ileum

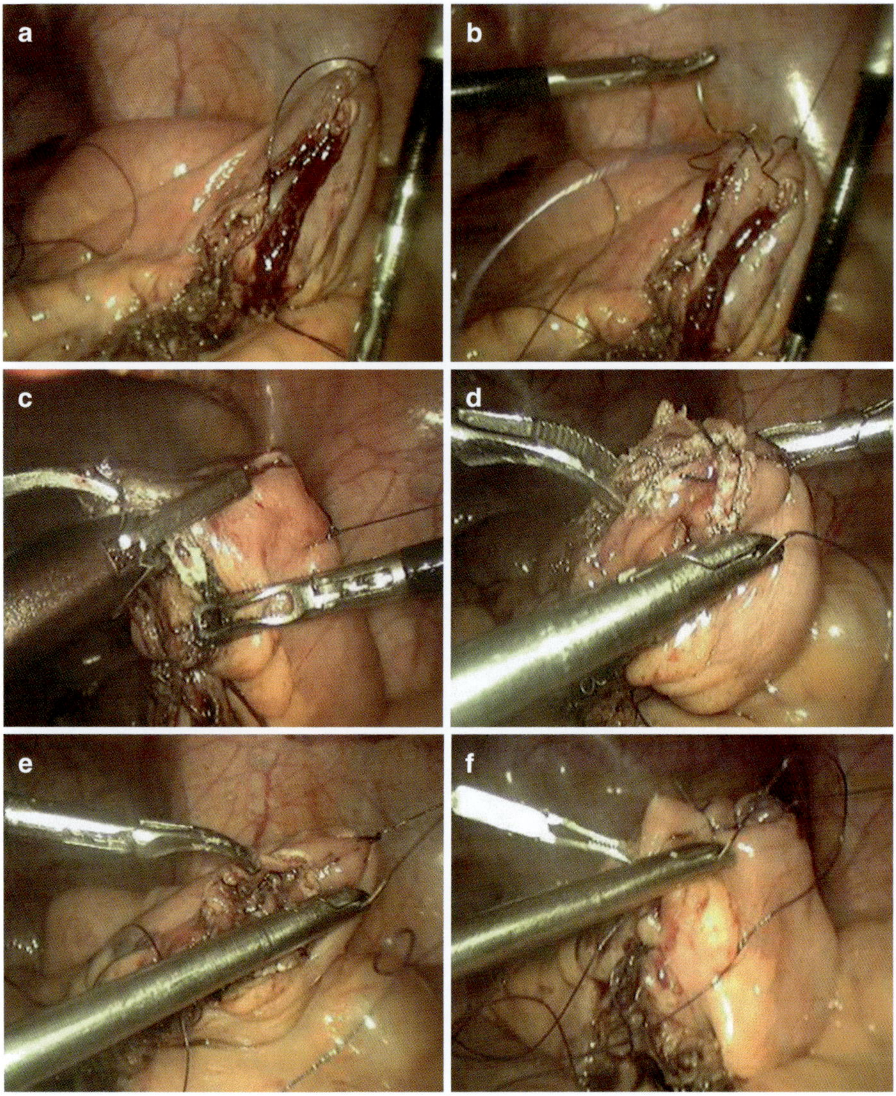

Fig. 4.93 Under the laparoscope, the two ends of the ileum are sutured and closed by traditional bowel anastomosis technique. (**a**) The ends of the two ilea are lifted up in the abdominal cavity and (**b**) suturing started at the posterior walls with the traditional bowel anastomosis technique (**c**) An ultrasonic scalpel is used to excise redundant tissues from the two closed ends of the ileum to open the ends (**d**, **e**) The two ends of the ilea are closed together with full-thickness interrupted sutures. (**f**) The seromuscular layers of both ilea are sutured by interrupted stitches

8. Creation of a new vagina: 10–20 ml of normal saline is injected in the tissue space between the urethra, bladder, and rectum. At the vaginal vestibular depression, a concave transverse incision is performed, followed by a blunt separation of the loose tissue between the urethra, the bladder, and the rectum to create a vaginal tunnel right up to the pelvic peritoneum (Fig. 4.95). An oval clamp is inserted through the vaginal vestibular incision till it reaches the pelvic peritoneum. Between the bladder and the rectum, there is an appropriate location for the pelvic vaginal opening (Fig. 4.96a); under the laparoscopic direct vision, a ultrasonic scalpel is used to open the pelvic peritoneum between the two heads of the oval clamp; this forms the new vaginal opening in the pelvis (Fig. 4.96b); this opening and the vaginal tunnel are further expanded to a sufficient width for vaginoplasty (Fig. 4.96c, d).

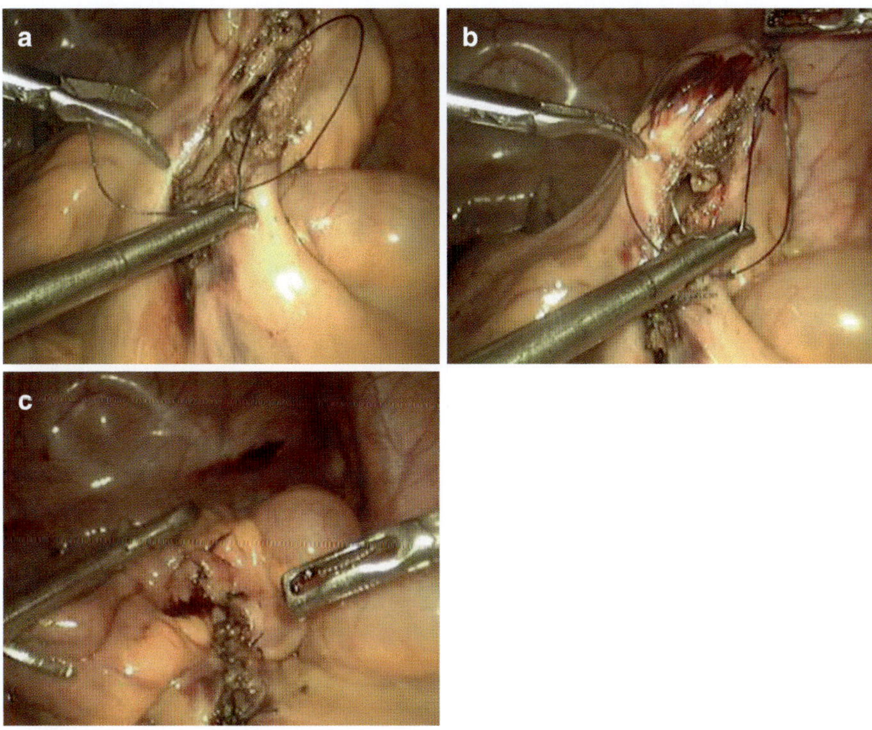

Fig. 4.94 The laparoscopic closure of the ileal mesentery by interrupted sutures. (**a**) starting to close the ileal mesentery from the proximal end (**b**) by continuous suturing closing the mesentery toward the ileum (**c**) careful inspection for any bleeding

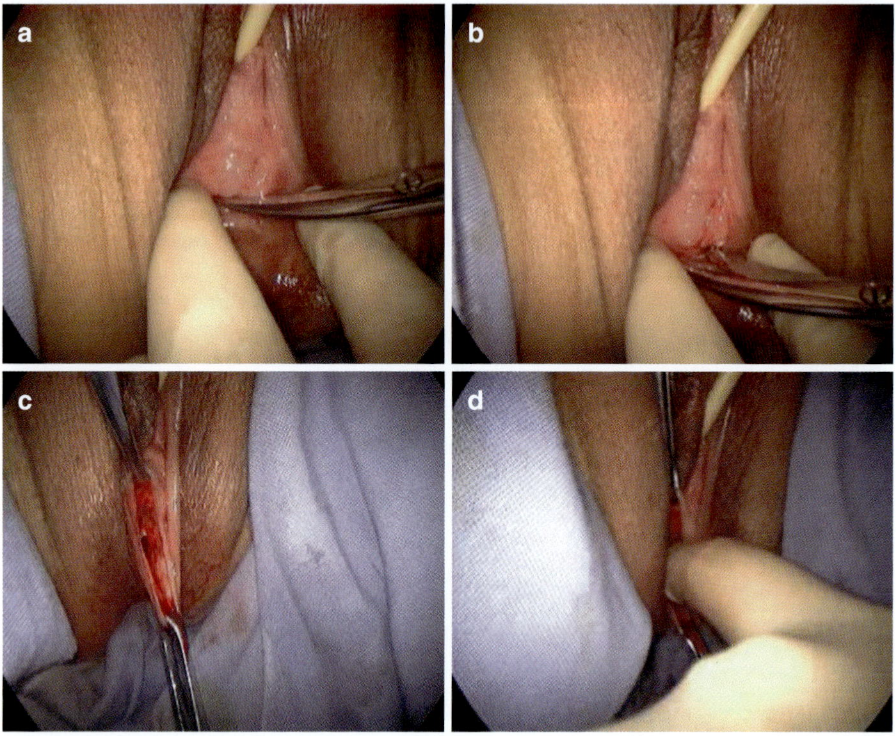

Fig. 4.95 Creation of a new vagina: (**a**) a transverse mucosal incision is made at the vaginal vestibule; (**b**) blunt separation of the loose tissue between the urethra, bladder, and rectum; (**c**) a vaginal tunnel is created with the vaginal mucosa pulled down to expose the vaginal opening; (**d**) digital examination to check the size of the vaginal tunnel

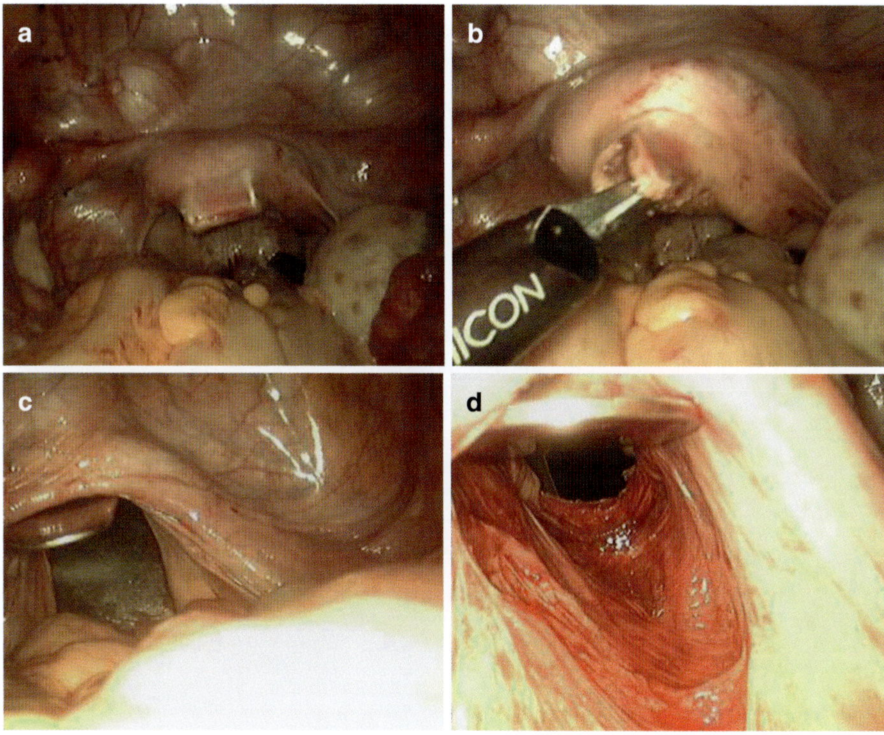

Fig. 4.96 The creation of pelvic vaginal opening under direct laparoscopic view: (**a**) a location for the pelvic vaginal stoma is selected. (**b**) A harmonic scalpel is to cut open the pelvic peritoneum between the two heads of an oval clamp. (**c**) The pelvic vaginal opening is further expanded to increase its size. (**d**) Vaginal inspection of the pelvic vaginal opening and the new vaginal tunnel

9. Transplantation of the isolated ileal loop and suturing it with the vestibular mucosa to form a new vagina: the remote end of the isolated ileal loop is pulled into the new vaginal tunnel (Fig. 4.97) and is sutured using 3/0 Dexon to the vaginal vestibular mucosa to form the new vaginal stoma. The top end of the transplanted ileal loop is fixed to the presacral region, so as to prevent any prolapse of the new vagina (Fig. 4.98). A vaginal mold is put into the ileal loop (Fig. 4.99).
10. Washing of pelvis and completion of the surgery: After surgery, the pelvis is cleaned and any blood clots removed. Hemostasis is observed. The blood supply at the anastomosis is checked for its good condition. Then the surgery is completed after taking out all surgical instruments, emptying any intraperitoneal CO_2 and closing all the abdominal wounds.

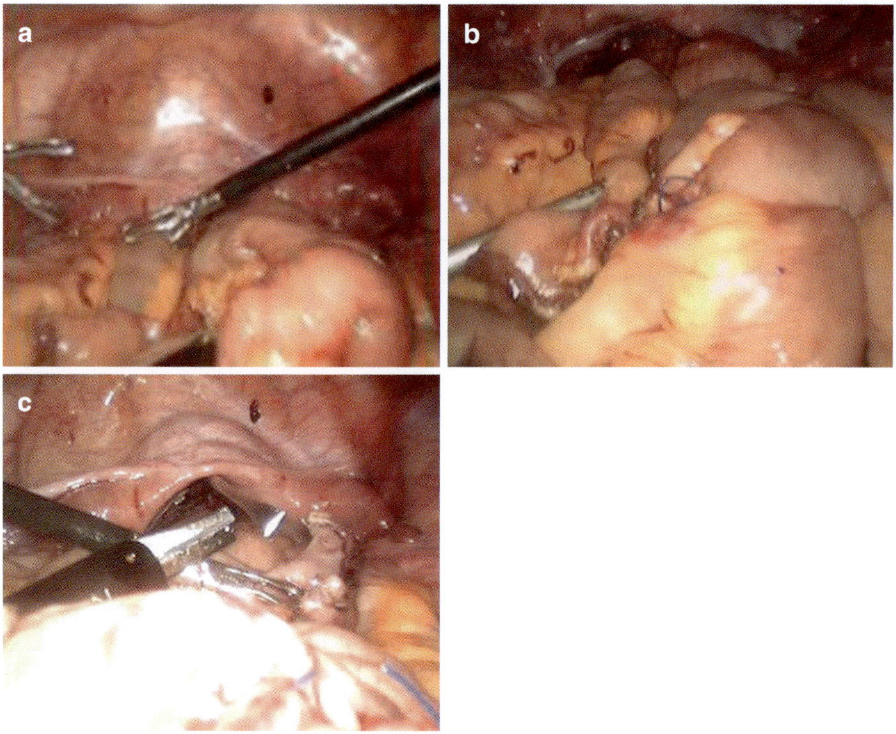

Fig. 4.97 The distal end of the transplant ileum is pushed down into the vaginal tunnel (**a**) the ends of the isolated ileal loop are identified (**b**) correct orientation to ensure good blood supply (**c**) pulling an end of the transplant ileum into the vaginal tunnel

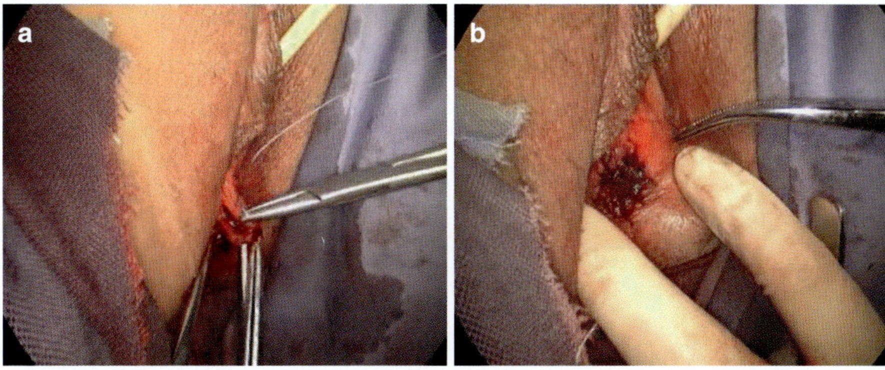

Fig. 4.98 (**a**) The distal end of the ileum is sutured to the vaginal vestibular mucosa (**b**) Inspection of the new vagina after the procedure was completed

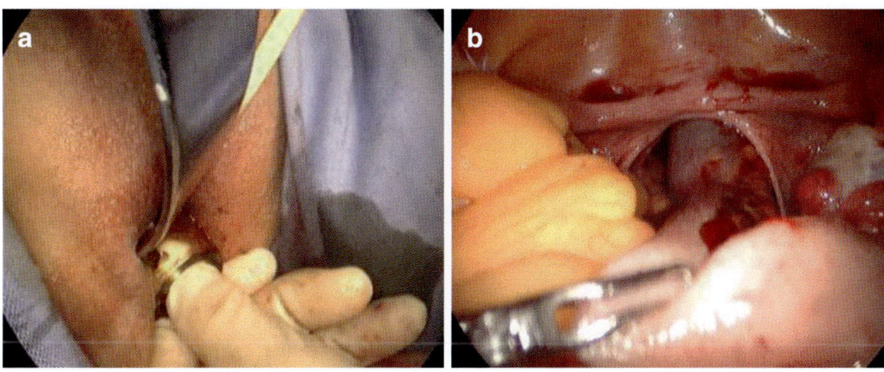

Fig. 4.99 (**a**) A vaginal mold is inserted into the transplant ileum (**b**) laparoscopic inspection of the new vagina and peritoneal cavity

Laparoscopic-assisted ileal vaginoplasty with minilaparotomy:

Under the direct vision of the laparoscope, the mesentery for the transplant ileal loop is isolated and freed by ultrasonic scalpel from the other mesentery. A suprapubic transverse minilaparotomy wound of 3–4 cm is then incised. The abdominal wound is opened layer by layer into the abdominal cavity (Fig. 4.100). Through this incision, the transplant ileal loop is pulled out of the abdominal cavity. Under direct vision, the transplant ileal loop is isolated and cut by endocutter. The two open ends of the ileum are then reanastomosed (Fig. 4.101) using No. 1 Vicryl sutures to suture with interrupted suturing of the full thickness of the two ends of the ileum (Figs. 4.101b, c) and then similarly for the seromuscular layers of the ileal wall (Fig. 4.101a, d). The transplant ileal loop with its closed ends and the remaining anastomosed ileum are put back into the abdominal cavity. The minilaparotomy wound will be closed. The remaining steps are the same as for the above total laparoscopic ileal vaginoplasty.

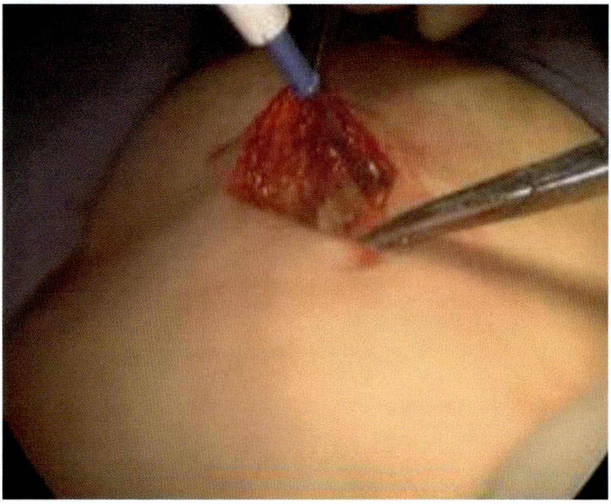

Fig. 4.100 A suprapubic minilaparotomy wound is performed

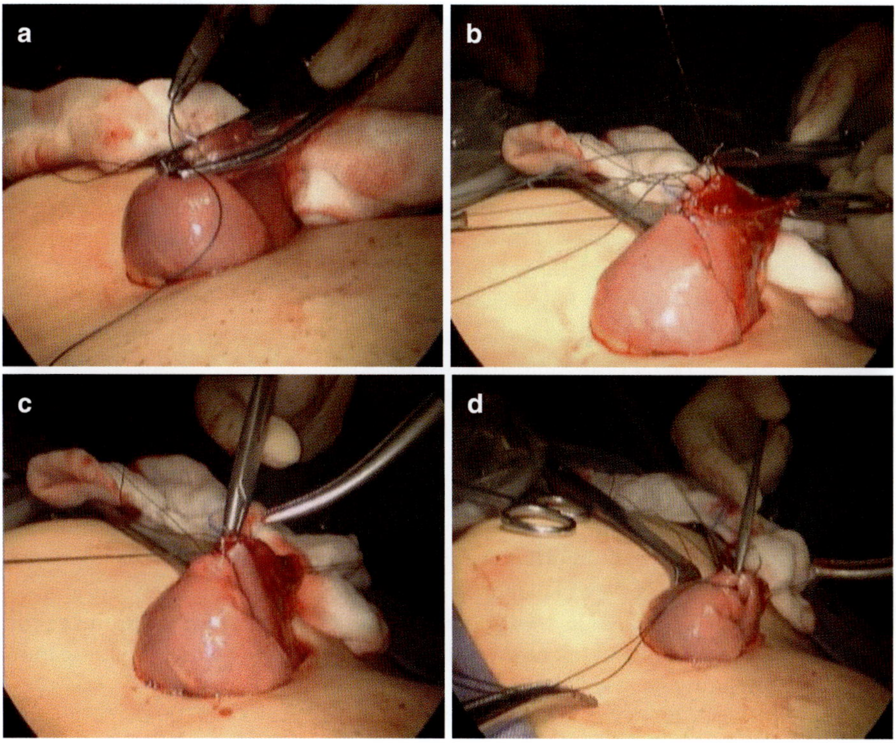

Fig. 4.101 The two open ends of the ileum are anastomosed by interrupted absorbable sutures in two layers: (**a**, **b**) full-thickness interrupted suturing, (**c**, **d**) interrupted seromuscular suturing

4.1.6.2 Surgical Techniques

1. Perform laparoscopic ileum resection and intestinal anastomosis, including the use of endocutter to excise the ileal loop and endocutter to perform functional anastomosis for the two open ends of the ileum and use of endoscopic suture technique for anastomosis on the open ends of the ileum and close the ileal mesentery, requiring higher technical requirements and physicians with skilled laparoscopic techniques.
2. Free the ileal mesentery sufficiently, or else the tension from dragging of the transplant to the pelvic to form a new vagina may become too large, but do not destroy too much of mesenteric vascular arch, keeping at least one vascular arch to ensure the survival of the intestinal transplant.
3. When dragging the remote end of the free ileal loop into the new vaginal tunnel hole for anastomosis with the vestibular mucosa, straighten out the free ileal loop to prevent twisting.
4. When making a tunnel for the new vagina, the vaginal vestibular mucosa is cut transversely after injecting 10–20 ml of normal saline with diluted pituitrin into the tissues between the urethra, bladder, and rectum. It is to expand the above tissue space and to reduce bleeding during the creation of the tunnel.
5. After separating the bladder and the rectum for some distance up to the pelvic peritoneum, the tunnel of the new vagina must be widened sufficiently to accommodate three fingers.

4.1.7 Laparoscopic-Assisted Sigmoid Vaginoplasty

Xianghua Huang

4.1.7.1 Anesthesia

General Anesthesia

1. Patient is in a lithotomy position, with routine vulval disinfection, surgical draping, and the insertion of indwelling catheter. Laparoscopy is performed via an umbilical incision and two operating ports at the left lower and right lower quadrant of the abdomen. After the trocars' placement, the operating table will be adjusted to 35 ° with a Trendelenburg position to facilitate the exposure of pelvic organs. A comprehensive assessment of abdominal and pelvic organs is first performed.
2. The sigmoid colon is then identified and exposed to show its mesentery and blood vessels. From the root of the mesenteric artery, ultrasonic scalpel is used to cut both the front and back peritoneum of the sigmoid mesentery, freeing it till reaching the pelvic peritoneum, while preserving the main mesenteric vessels to the sigmoid colon. The upper and lower ends of mesentery to the sigmoid colon are set free.
3. At the depression of the vaginal vestibule, a transverse incision is made and the space of loose tissues between bladder and rectum is bluntly separated horizontally to form a new vaginal tunnel. Under the laparoscopic vision, a 12 mm trocar was inserted through the vaginal tunnel. A linear endo-stapler is introduced via the trocar and used to cut and close the lower part of the sigmoid colon.
4. A 4 cm long abdominal incision is made at the left lower quadrant of the abdomen, through which the sigmoid colon is delivered out of the abdominal cavity. A segment of 8–12 cm sigmoid colon with its blood supply will be isolated and cut out for its use in the sigmoid vaginoplasty. Both ends of the transplant sigmoid colon are closed with interrupted sutures and are delivered back into the abdominal cavity for later use. The other proximal end of the cut sigmoid colon will be closed with absorbable purse-string sutures, but a circular stapler head is inserted and tied with this end of the sigmoid colon. This proximal end of the sigmoid colon is also returned into the abdominal cavity for anastomosis to the distal end of the sigmoid colon. The abdominal wound is now closed with sutures layer by layer.
5. A circular stapler with staples is inserted into the distal end of the sigmoid colon through the anus and joined firmly with the circular stapler head at the proximal end of the sigmoid colon. Attention is paid to make sure the two ends of the colon mesenteries are corresponding. Then the stapler trigger is pulled and fired to complete the anastomosis of the sigmoid colon. The stapler is then removed through the anus. Both sides of the bowel tissue which the stapler cut through are checked. Each stump of tissue should consist of a complete and continuous loop of bowel tissues.

6. The perineal trocar is now removed. With blunt dissection, the vaginal tunnel is further enlarged in the space between the urinary bladder and rectum, forming a tunnel of 4 cm in diameter. The other reserved transplant sigmoid colon segment with its vascular pedicle will be dragged through the new vaginal tunnel to the vaginal opening at the introitus. The closed end of the sigmoid colon is now opened and then both the sigmoid colon mucosa and vaginal vestibular mucosa are sutured together with absorbable sutures. A soft vaginal mold is inserted to the new vagina and fixed in position. Laparoscopic examination is performed to examine the colon anastomosis and confirm that there is no tension or abnormal bowel color. Laparoscope and cannulas are now removed, and the portal wounds are closed to complete the surgery.

4.1.7.2 Single-Port Laparoscopic-Assisted Sigmoid Vaginoplasty

A single-port device consisting of multiple ports is inserted into an umbilical incision of 2.5 cm (Fig. 4.102). After pneumoperitoneum is established, a 5 or 10 mm 30° laparoscope and other semirigid curved instruments are introduced into the abdominal cavity. After a thorough abdominal examination (Figs. 4.103 and 4.104), an ultrasonic scalpel is used to free the sigmoid colon and divide the mesenteric peritoneum (Fig. 4.105). A linear cutter is now inserted via a 12 mm trocar through the vaginal tunnel to cut (Fig. 4.106) and closed off from the distal end of the sigmoid colon (Fig. 4.107).

A sigmoid colon segment with adequate blood supply from its vascular arch is identified. This segment is about 8–12 cm long and is now cut off by a linear endocutter to prepare for the vaginal transplant. After that, the blood flow and colon color from the edges of the cut sigmoid colon are observed. The single-port device is now removed from the umbilical incision, and this segment of the sigmoid colon is dragged through the umbilical incision. A purse-string suturing with an absorbable suture is performed to close the end of the sigmoid colon and fix a circular stapler head into this proximal end (Fig. 4.108). Similar to the above laparoscopic sigmoid vaginoplasty procedure, a circular stapler with staples is inserted into the distal end of the sigmoid colon through the anus and joined firmly with the circular stapler head at the proximal end of sigmoid colon. Then the stapler trigger is fired to complete the anastomosis. The stapler is then removed through the anus (Fig. 4.109). The reserved sigmoid colon with its vascular pedicle is then dragged through the new vaginal tunnel (Fig. 4.110), and the procedure will be similar to that of laparoscopic-assisted sigmoid vaginoplasty.

4.1.7.3 Postoperative Management

The soft vaginal mold is removed at 3–5 days after the surgery depending on the patients' recovery. The new vagina is flushed clean and a hard vaginal mold is used to replace the soft mold. The urinary catheter can now be removed. Patients will be guided to perform vaginal douching and continuous to use the vaginal mold for 3 months. Depending on the sexual life of patients, intermittent vaginal dilatation may be necessary.

4.1.7.4 Surgical Techniques

1. It is important to observe the vascular arch to ensure adequate blood supply and survival of the transplant sigmoid colon. The sigmoid mesentery should be adequately freed and mobilized so the transplant colon is not under tension when it is pushed down to the pelvis to form the vagina. If the mesentery is adequately free and mobilized, it would be preferably to rotate the colon 180 ° in the transplant position. Hopefully, the reverse peristalsis of the transplanted colon segment can reduce postoperative "vaginal" secretions and prevent vaginal prolapse due to its reverse peristaltic movement.
2. When the sigmoid colon mucosa is sutured with vaginal vestibular mucosa, it is important to straighten the colonic mesentery in the right direction and make sure the sigmoid colon segment is not twisted.
3. Intraoperative dilatation of the vaginal tunnel to a diameter of 4 cm is important as well as postoperative teaching for patients to continue vaginal dilatation according to their sex activities.
4. Single-port laparoscopic surgery has the problems of narrow spaces between surgical instruments, leading to easy clashing and increasing the difficulty of the operation. It might be necessary to make another accessory port, at no additional damage but reducing the difficulty of operation. Single-port laparoscopic sigmoid vaginoplasty is technically demanding. The surgeon requires plenty of clinical experience and laparoscopic surgical skills to complete a successful single-port laparoscopic procedure.

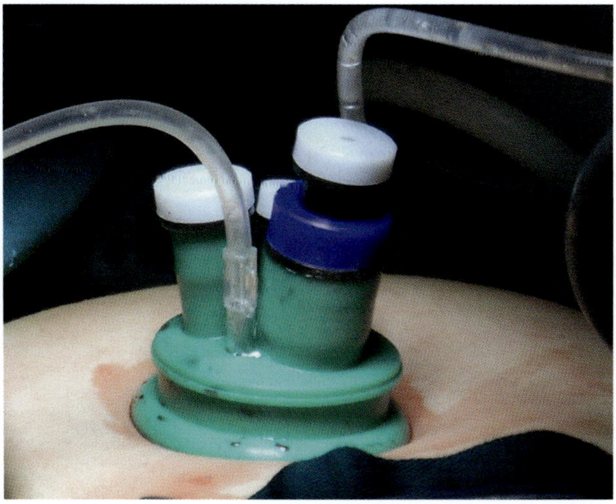

Fig. 4.102 A single-port device with multiple ports is inserted at the umbilical incision

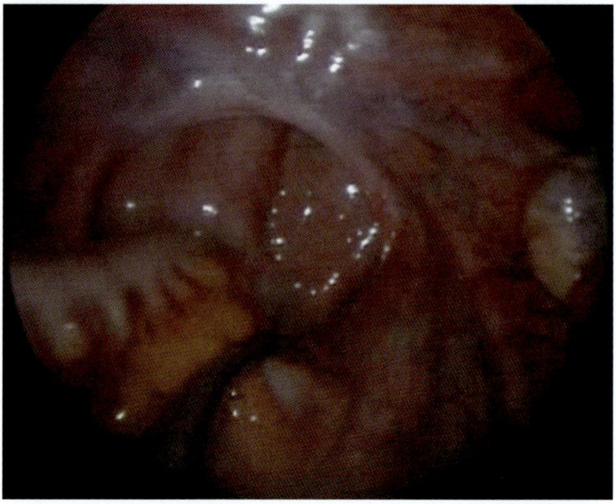

Fig. 4.103 Examination of the pelvic cavity: the ovaries and uterus are absent. Both fallopian tubes are normal

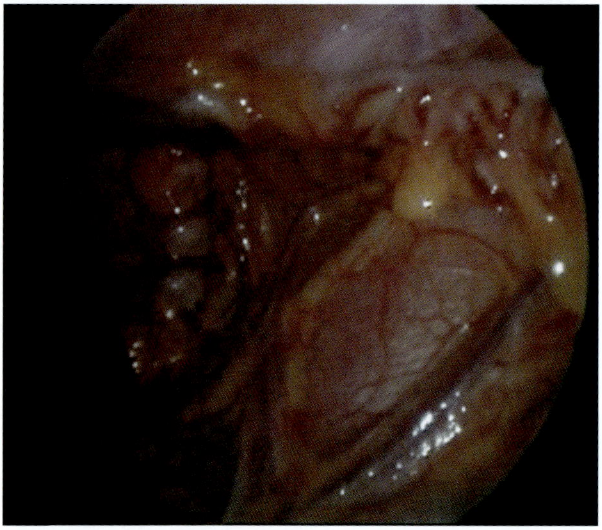

Fig. 4.104 Examination of the sigmoid colon in the pelvic cavity, showing the mesentery and its vascular arch

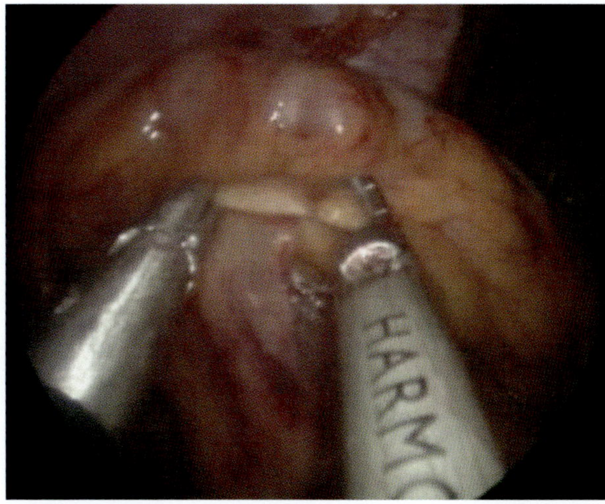

Fig. 4.105 Harmonic scalpel is used to free the sigmoid colon

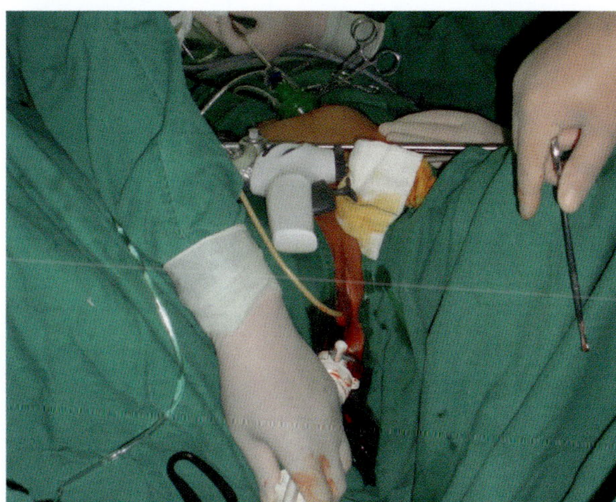

Fig. 4.106 A 12 mm trocar is inserted through the new vaginal tunnel, followed by the insertion of a linear cutter and stapler

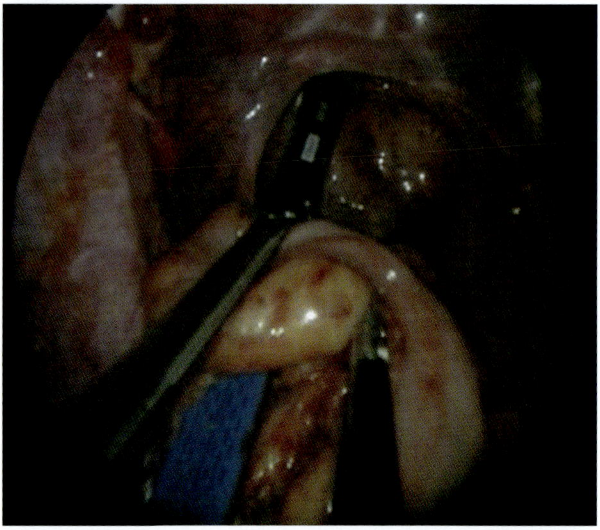

Fig. 4.107 A linear cutter and stapler cut and close the distal end of the sigmoid colon

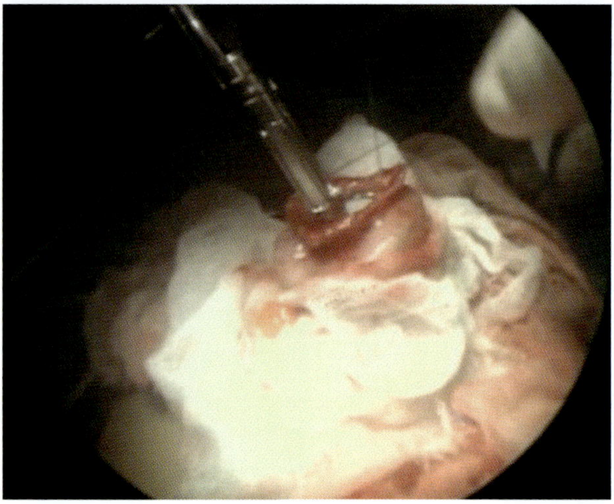

Fig. 4.108 A circular staple head is inserted into the proximal ends of the sigmoid colon and closed with a purse-string suture

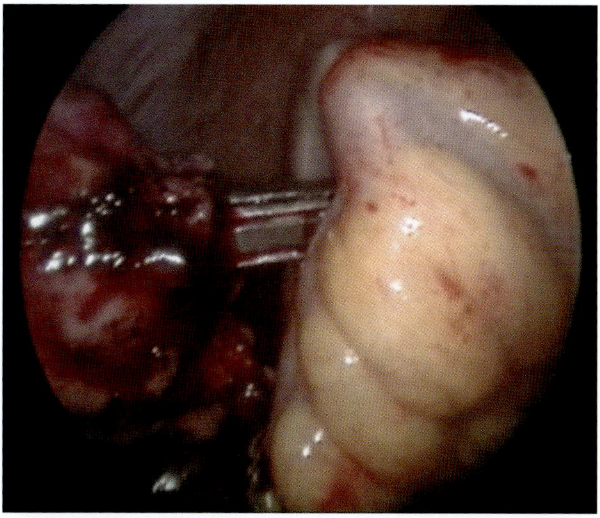

Fig. 4.109 Anastomosis of both ends of the sigmoid colon

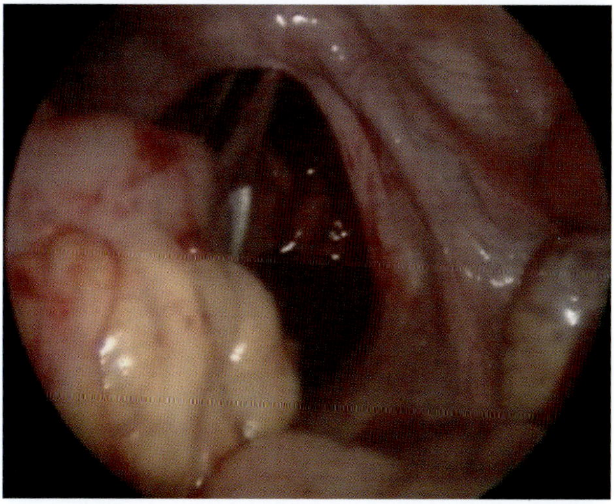

Fig. 4.110 Dragging down the reserved transplant sigmoid colon together with its vascular pedicle through the vaginal tunnel

4.1.8 Vaginoplasty with Tissue Engineering Biological Patch

Huimei Zhou and Lan Zhu

Anesthesia: Intravenous, epidural, or general anesthesia can be used for this surgery.

4.1.8.1 Surgical Procedures

Materials

Biological patch, a dermal matrix material, is obtained by using applied tissue engineering technology which decellularizes human corpse tissues to obtain an extracellular matrix. It retains the extracellular matrix and a three-dimensional frame structure and is a dermal substitute. Our hospital is currently using a biological patch from porcine small intestinal submucosa (Surgisis®, Cook Medical, Bloomington, IN, USA). The specifications of the patch are 10×8 cm in sizes, preserved with sterile saline at 4 °C (Fig. 4.111).

Preparation of Biological Patch

A biological patch with sizes 10×8 cm is used. It is made into a cylinder tube sewn on its edges with interrupted 3/0 Dexon sutures, but closed on one end and the other end opened. The length of the cylinder is 10 cm long, and its cylinder surface is cut with several longitudinal incisions of about 0.5–1 cm to facilitate drainage (Fig. 4.112).

Creation of a Vaginal Tunnel for a New Vagina

The bladder is emptied with a urinary catheter which is left indwelling to serve as a guide to reduce bladder injury. The vaginal vestibule is then incised transversely for 2 cm in length. The space between the bladder and the rectum is separated bluntly with fingers to a depth of 9–10 cm. During the digital separation, rectal examination can be performed to serve as a guide to reduce rectal injury. It is important to perform adequate hemostasis and washing with saline to ensure no active bleeding in the vaginal tunnel (Fig. 4.113).

Preparation of Seedling Cells from the Vaginal Vestibular Mucosa

Clip a small piece of tissue from the vaginal vestibular mucosa, cut it up into smaller pieces, and scatter them as seedling cells onto the prepared biological patch (Fig. 4.114).

Implanting and Fixing the Biological Patch

A cylinder made from the biological patch is now sutured at three points transversely using 1/0 Vicryl sutures to the top end of the new vagina. Additional sutures are sewn to the middle, the left, and the right side to fix the biological patches to the new vagina. More interrupted sutures are used to fix the open end of biological patch to the vaginal vestibular opening. Sterile surgical gauzes are put inside two overlaying condoms to form a soft mold to fill the new vagina tightly and as far as possible without any loose space (Figs. 4.115, 4.116, and 4.117).

Closing the Vaginal Opening

The new vaginal opening is now closed with interrupted No. 7 silk suture to close the bilateral labia majora so as to keep the soft mold inside the new vagina. At the end of surgery, digital rectal examination should be performed to check if there is any rectal injury. An indwelling urinary catheter is often necessarily used for a long time.

Postoperative Management

On the tenth day after operation, the soft mold is taken out from the vagina and the urinary catheter is removed. A silicone mold to replace the soft mold is now used for at least 3 months depending on the condition of the vagina and the patient's sex life. The patient may have to use a mold or continually expand the vagina by herself if it is necessary.

Key Technical Points

1. There should be adequate hemostasis at the surgery. As far as possible, there should also be a tight fit between the biological patch and the surrounding tissue of the new vaginal tunnel. It is to allow easier spreading of epithelial cells onto the tissue, to have a better chance of survival. At the end, the biological patch can be epithelialized and replaced by the new mucosal epithelium.
2. During the surgery, the vaginal vestibular mucosa cells are used as seedling cells which are scattered onto the biological patch. This hopefully will speed up the epithelialization process after the vaginoplasty using the biological patch.
3. Biological patches have convenient sources. Using biological patch, the body damage and suffering caused by autologous transplant can also be avoided. The heterogeneous source of biological patch should be the direction of future development, with a vast potential for commercialization and stock supplies.

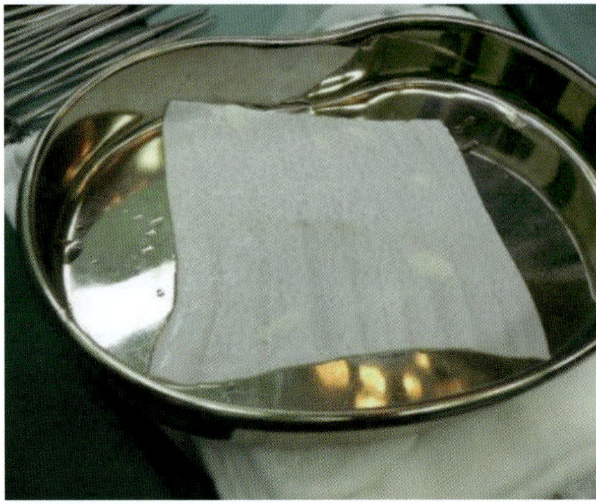

Fig. 4.111 Biological patch

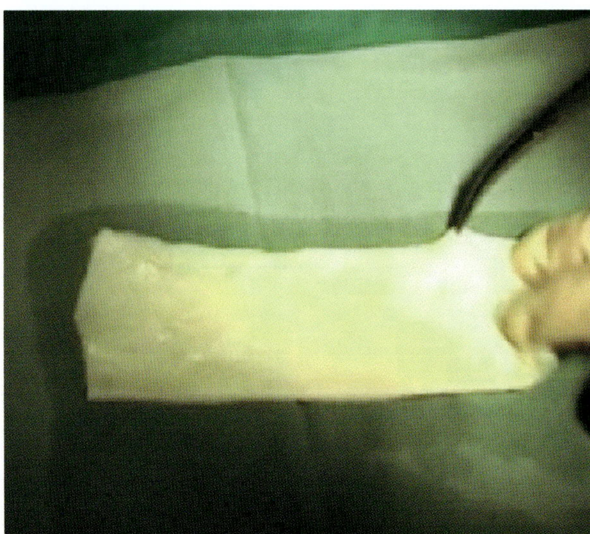

Fig. 4.112 Biological patch sutured into a cylindrical shape

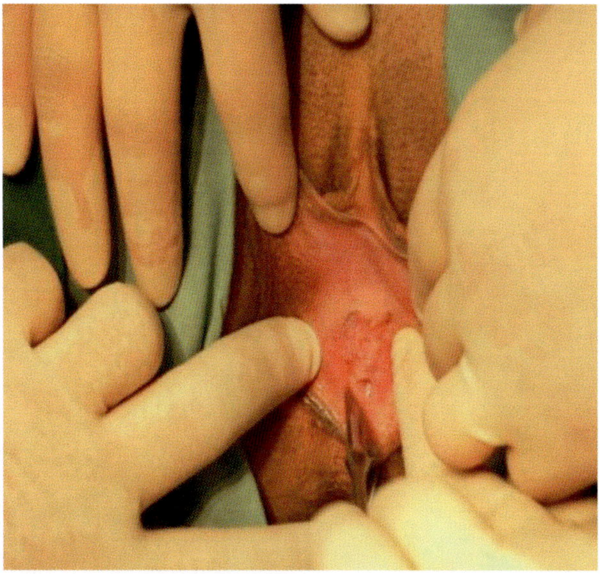

Fig. 4.113 Making a tunnel for the new vagina

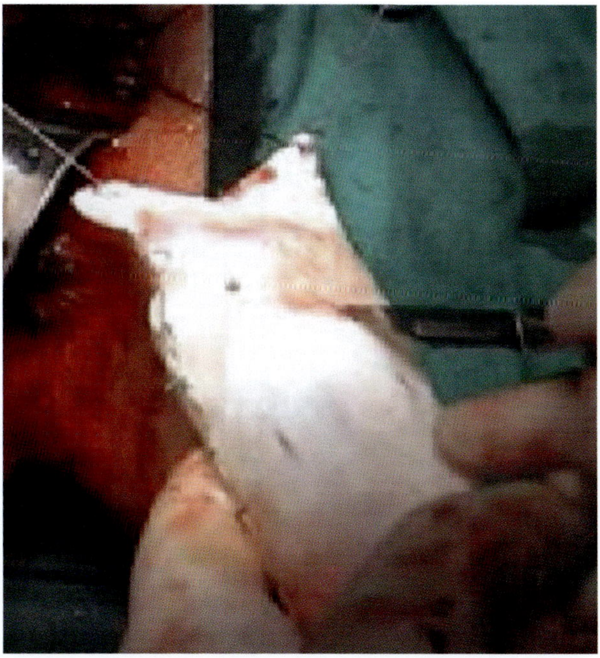

Fig. 4.114 The cylindrical surface has longitudinal incisions for drainage and is scattered with the seedling cells of vaginal vestibular mucosa

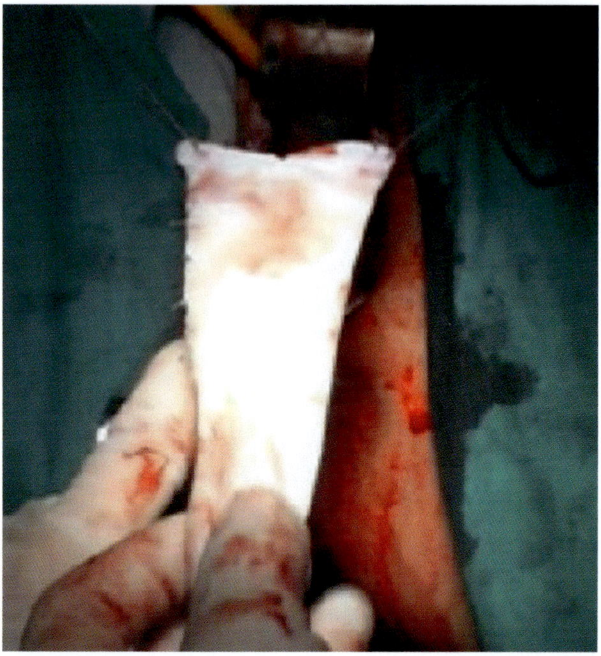

Fig. 4.115 Implanting the biological patch

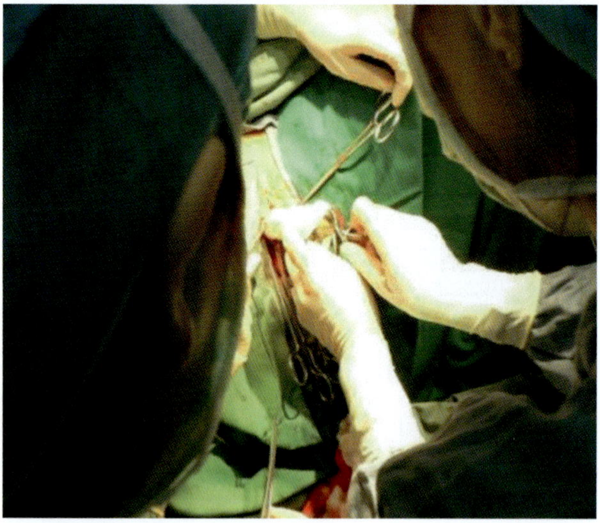

Fig. 4.116 Inserting the soft vaginal mold

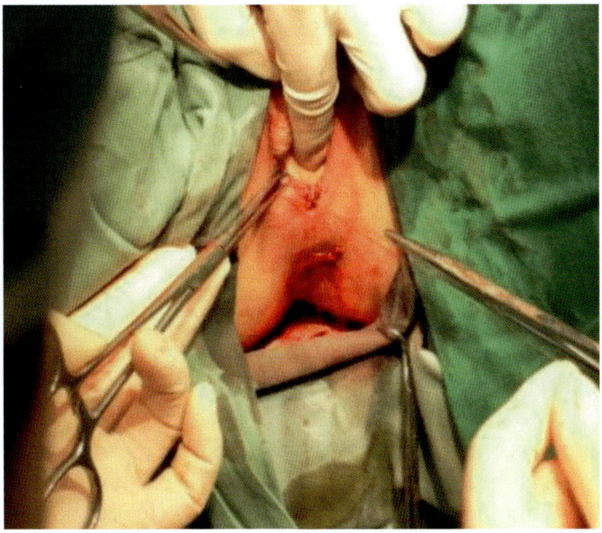

Fig. 4.117 Fixing the vaginal patch and closing the vaginal opening

4.2 Vaginal Atresia

Jie Yang and Lan Zhu

4.2.1 Overview

4.2.1.1 The Concept, Embryology, and Anatomical Classification of Vaginal Atresia

Vaginal atresia refers to a normal uterus with complete or partial vaginal atresia anomalies, associated or not associated with cervical anomaly. This group of patients often has a functioning uterine endometrium.

Although there are some descriptions on the embryological and anatomical basis of vaginal atresia, there are many controversies without standardization. The most popular theory is that the vagina is developed from the sinovaginal bulb of the urogenital sinus and the primordial vagina (fusion of the paramesonephric ducts). The upper 1/3 to 4/5 epithelium of the vaginal lumen is formed from the primordial vagina and that of the lower 2/3 to 1/5 epithelium from sinovaginal bulb (Fig. 4.118). In 1976, Simpson proposed that vaginal atresia is different from congenital absence of vagina. The former is caused by developmental defects of the urogenital sinus, and the uterus is usually normal, but possibly combined with cervical anomaly; the latter is the result of abnormal development of the paramesonephric ducts, with absence of uterus and vagina (Fig. 4.119). The incidence of congenital absence of vagina is 1/4000 to 1/5000, of which only 7–8 % were vaginal atresia associated with normal uterus. Therefore, those without a vagina are mostly congenital absence of vagina and uterus, only a small number are complete vaginal atresia.

Depending on length of vaginal atresia and cervical development, vaginal atresia can be divided into complete and partial vaginal atresia. So, the Beijing Union Medical College Hospital has divided vaginal atresia into two types based on their anatomical characteristics: type I – lower vaginal atresia, but with a normal development of the upper vagina, cervix, and uterus and may be regarded as a developmental defect of the urogenital sinus (Fig. 4.120); type II – a complete atresia of the vagina, often associated with cervical anomaly. The uterus is normal or may be with anomaly, but the endometrium is always functional. It can be considered as the absence of developmental differentiation into vaginal sinus, vaginal cord, and vaginal plate (Fig. 4.121).

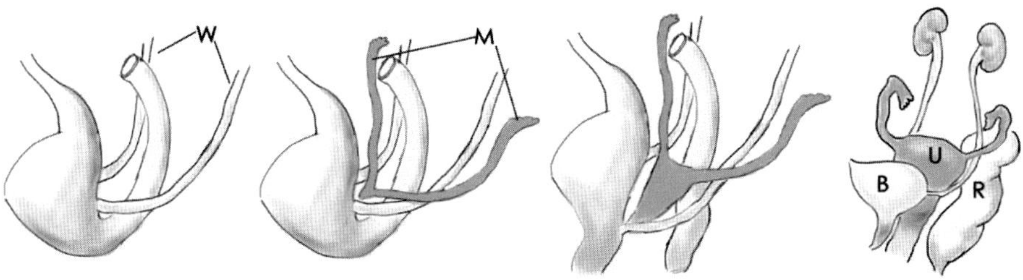

Fig. 4.118 The development of the vagina. *W* Wolffian duct, *M* paramesonephric duct, *B* bladder, *U* uterus, *R* rectum

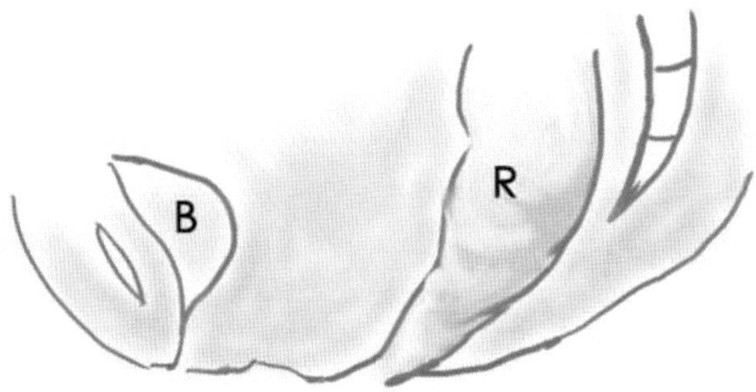

Fig. 4.119 Congenital absence of vagina. *B* bladder, *R* rectum

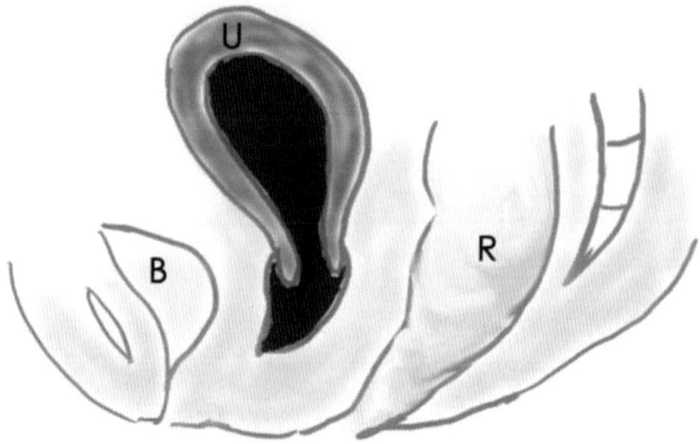

Fig. 4.120 Type I vaginal atresia. *B* bladder, *U* uterus, *R* rectum

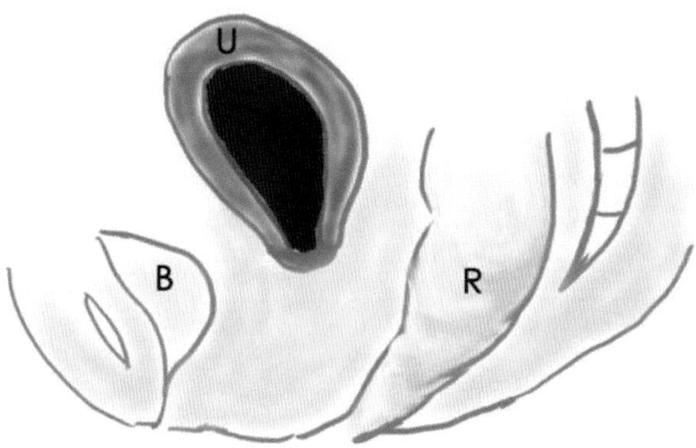

Fig. 4.121 Type II vaginal atresia. *B* bladder, *U* uterus, *R* rectum

4.2.1.2 Key Diagnostic Points

Vaginal atresia belongs to obstructive reproductive tract disorders, with onset at puberty. The main features are primary amenorrhea, cyclical abdominal pain, and pelvic mass. The onset of symptoms and severity are related to the functioning endometrium. Those of vaginal atresia type I have normal uterus and functioning endometrium. Therefore, symptoms appear earlier and are more severe. Medical consultations are often timely. The clinical findings are distended upper vagina with blood clots, and in severe cases, there is blood retention in the cervix and uterine cavity. On examination, a pelvic mass can be found in the lower pelvis, above the vaginal atresia, and in front of the rectum. Due to earlier medical consultation, the menstrual blood can be timely drained. Menstrual blood reflux into the fallopian tubes and pelvic endometriosis is uncommon. For type II vaginal atresia, they are often associated with cervical anomaly. Menstrual blood can easily reflux through the fallopian tubes into the pelvis and thus increasing the chance of hematosalpinx and endometriosis. This group of patients does not usually have an upper vaginal mass, and rectal examination often does not show a mass in front of the rectum. However, sometimes there might be excessive retention of blood clots forming an upper vaginal mass, making it difficult to distinguish the two types of vaginal atresia. Therefore, preoperative imaging assessment with MRI and ultrasound scan is very important.

4.2.2 Surgical Indications

Vaginal atresia is an obstructive reproductive tract anomaly. Surgery is the main treatment. Once diagnosed, surgery should be scheduled.

4.2.3 Timing of Surgery

Patient with type I vaginal atresia has a pelvic mass above the atresia, making it easier to locate the lesion. The distended vaginal wall can also provide adequate mucosa, resulting in a higher success rate. If the patients do not have obvious contraindications for surgery, the vaginal atresia can be treated directly. Type II vaginal atresia surgery is different from many other gynecologic surgeries. The surgery should be performed at the time of severe menstrual symptoms at the time of excessive blood retention because the lesion can be more easily identified and the anatomical structure is clearer. Therefore, the risk of bladder and rectum injury can be reduced.

4.2.4 Preoperative Preparation

Patient should fast overnight and has enema for bowel preparation before operation.

4.2.5 Key Technical Points

According to the type of vaginal atresia, the treatments are different.

4.2.5.1 Type I Vaginal Atresia

The surgery aims to remove the obstruction, i.e., to incise the closed segment of the vagina, so as to open up the upper vagina to drain the retained menstrual blood. The key point of surgery is to obtain the correct surgical direction to avoid damage to the urethra or rectum. If necessary, ultrasound monitoring at the time of the surgery will help to ensure the orientation. Generally, the surgery is chosen to be operated at the time of a menstrual period. Firstly, a needle puncture which can draw out blood will reveal the direction of surgical incision. Then the closed space between the urethra and rectum is incised and expanded inward as far as possible until a cavity with blood clots is reached. The blood is drained. For vaginal atresia type I, the operation is more difficult than the imperforate hymen and the transverse vaginal septum. Similar to the technique of puncture-cut-drainage (P-C-D) approach, the surgery should follow the observations of "five words guidelines" of puncture, cut, expand, drain, and trim (Fig. 4.122).

Puncture – The prominent cystic and bulging part of the vaginal mass should be selected by palpation and marked with a finger accurately. The finger is inserted into the rectum to guide the surgery to avoid rectal injury. A 16 G needle is inserted while maintaining a gently suction after piercing the cystic mass. If there is no content on suction, the needle is withdrawn back and forth till blood content can be obtained. Then the location and direction are identified and locked on for further surgery. Only with an accurate puncture, the tissue can be cut and separated accurately. If the puncture is inaccurate, the cut can go astray causing injury to adjacent organs.

Cut – Preferably a small sharp knife is used to cut along the puncture needle until blood is visible. The knife is then kept in place, followed by inserting a long curved vascular forceps forward until it is clearly inside the cystic cavity. That procedure will be considered successful.

Expand – That is the step to expand the wound, to achieve adequate drainage of the blood clots. A vascular forceps is used assisted by further cutting with the knife to expand the wound.

Drain – Adequate expansion and exposure are required to achieve a complete drainage.

Trim – Excessive tissues of the vaginal atresia are trimmed to prevent adhesion. The vaginal vestibular mucosa can now be pushed into the new vaginal space and sutured to the upper vaginal mucosa with absorbable sutures.

If the obliterated area of the vaginal atresia type I is short, the wound gap will be small, then the vestibular mucosa can be pushed over the wound and sutured to the vaginal mucosa easily; this can be a more effective surgery. After the surgery, there will be no longer any menstruation and sex problems. For individual patient with vaginal stenosis after operation, a vaginal mold should be used and digital dilatation of the vagina performed regularly. Before a complete epithelialization of the vaginal wound surface, a vaginal mold should always be used. Afterward, a vaginal mold can be used intermittently until marriage.

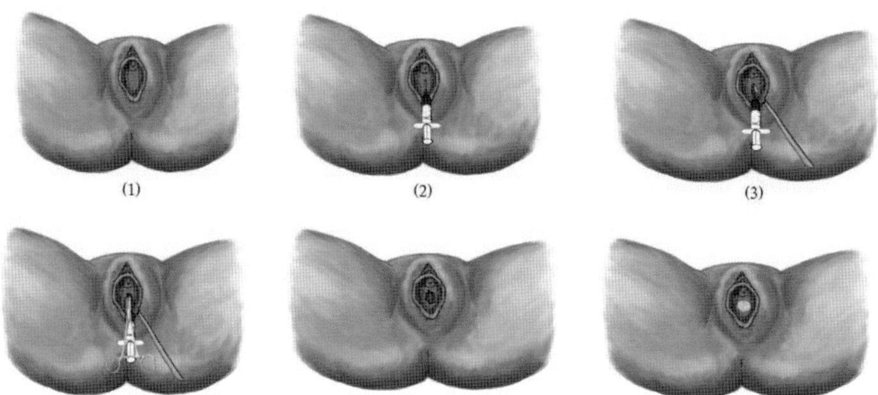

(1) (2) (3)
(4) (5) (6)

Fig. 4.122 Type I vaginal atresia surgery. (**1**) Vaginal atresia with no vagina (**2**) Puncture at the bulging part (**3**) Cut along the puncture needle (**4**) Expand the wound and drain all blood clots (**5**) Trim excessive tissue to enlarge the wound (**6**) Insertion of a vaginal mold

4.2.5.2 Type II Vaginal Atresia

The key issue of treatment is whether to keep the uterus. If not, it will be relatively simple to have a hysterectomy to relieve the symptom and to perform an artificial vagina surgery at the same time or before marriage. Hysterectomy is recommended for the following conditions: (1) uterine morphology and function will not become normal after the surgery, (2) anticipating cervical readhesions after cervicoplasty, and (3) severe uterine and fallopian tube infection. At present for suitable patients, it is recommended that the conservative treatment should be offered to retain the uterus, so as to provide opportunities for future reproduction. Some authors recommend for patients with type II vaginal atresia a laparoscopic examination to evaluate the uterine development in the pelvis. With a developed uterus with no anomaly, no or mild pelvic endometriosis, one could consider a vaginoplasty, cervicoplasty, and reconnection operation. Some scholars also advocate the suppression of menstruations, to facilitate the vaginoplasty surgery, followed by cervicoplasty after the complete epithelization of the new vagina. However, as reported in the literature, even after this conservative treatment of the vaginal atresia, the chance of pregnancy is extremely rare. So far only six cases of successful pregnancy had been reported in the literature, the majority of patients eventually have to remove the uterus. For patients with cervical anomaly and without cardinal ligaments and uterosacral ligaments, even if pregnant, they are prone to have adverse pregnancy outcomes. Therefore, the consensus is to advocate hysterectomy for these patients.

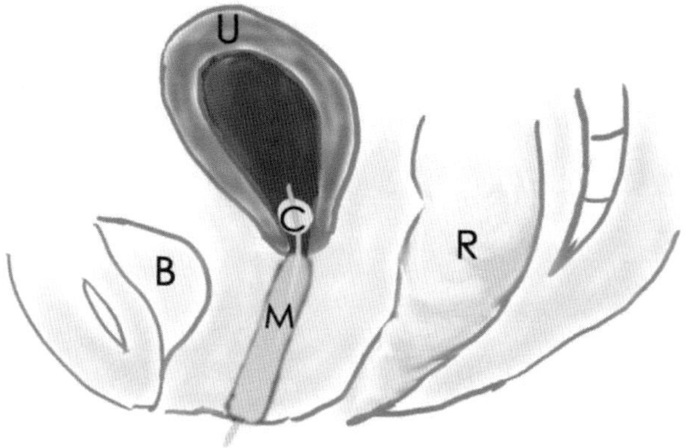

Fig. 4.123 Surgery for type II vaginal atresia. *B* bladder, *U* uterus, *R* rectum, *C* catheter; *M* mold

For type II vaginal atresia, the "open up" procedure is very difficult because the direction of puncture and incision is not easy to master. The tissue space between the urethra, bladder, and rectum is not as loose and easily separated as for the congenital absence of vagina. It is also difficult to obtain any blood content with a needle puncture because the blood in the "top end" is less, and the sac is ill defined. Even when a new vagina is "created," it is also vulnerable for readhesion; besides, the cervix is also not well developed; it still has difficulty to reconnect to the uterus. This requires an anastomosis procedure for the upper uterus and lower vagina together with a cervicoplasty. Sometimes the vaginal mucosa, labia minora, and skin flap can be used as reconstruction materials (Fig. 4.123). Some surgeons may also use pelvic peritoneum performed by the laparoscopic vaginoplasty approach for patients with type II vaginal atresia.

After cervicoplasty, it is important to place some support at the right place in the cervical canal. Reports in the literature proposed that iodoform gauze, Foley catheter, or closed thoracic drainage tube can be used. Iodoform gauze used after surgery not only can prevent wound adhesion, but also reduce the risk of infection. However, it can easily fall off. Foley catheter can be used effectively to provide continuous support to the cervix, but during the water injection to distend the Foley's balloon. Its location is hard to control because it can easily shift off and is difficult to reach and keep at the predetermined position during the surgery. Postoperative ultrasonic examination is required regularly to review the location of the water balloon. Yet, it can still fall off easily.

Grand D reported the use of a self-expanding nickel-titanium alloy-coated metallic stent in the cervix in a difficult and severe recurrent cervical stenosis (Figs. 4.124 and 4.125). Such stent is widely used in interventional vascular stent therapy. The stent was removed after 9 months. During the time with stent placement and 2 months after removal of the stent, there were normal menstruations without any complications. In his patients, 2 months after stent removal, pregnancy was successful. Therefore, Grand D reckoned that placing a coated stent into the cervix could be an effective way to preserve fertility in patients with recurrent cervical stenosis.

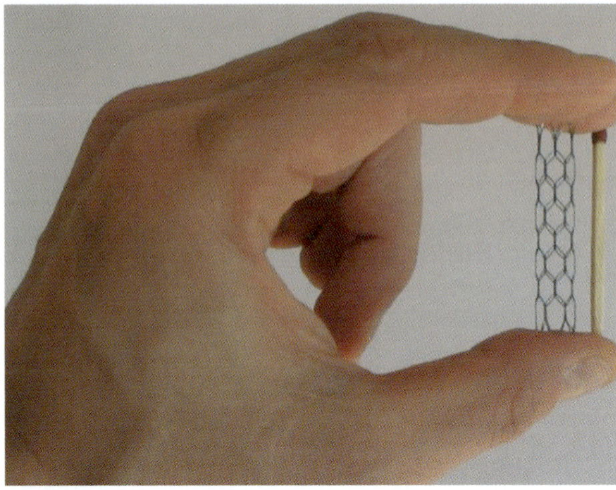

Fig. 4.124 The application of a nickel-titanium-coated vascular stent as the cervical stent in cervicoplasty

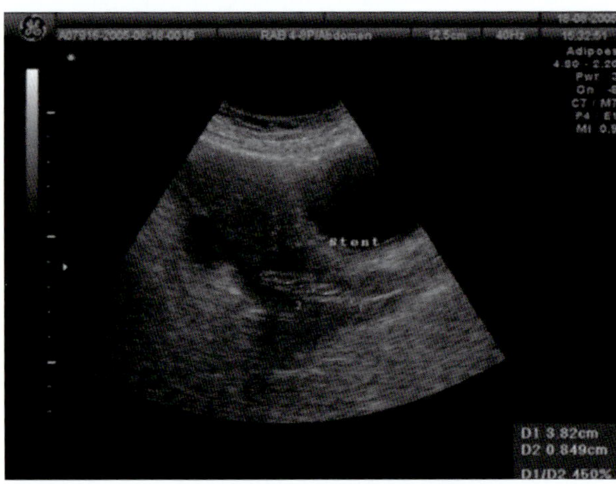

Fig. 4.125 Ultrasound scan shows a cervical stent in the cervical canal

4.3 Transverse Vaginal Septum

Xianghua Huang and Qiushi Wang

Transverse vaginal septum is formed after the ends of the paramesonephric ducts fail to connect completely or only partially connect with the urogenital sinus. The incidence of this disorder among the general population is 1:30,000–80,000. The majority of patients are not discovered and diagnosed at birth, childhood, and puberty. The septum can be located in any part of the vagina, but most commonly, it is in the upper one third of the vagina. Those located at the lower vagina has to be differentiated from the imperforate hymen. Transverse vaginal septum can be a single septum, but it may also be multiple septa. It can be associated with longitudinal vaginal septum, cervical atresia, hypoplastic uterus, urinary tract anomaly, skeletal malformation, and anomalies in other parts of the body. Whether it is a complete or incomplete transverse septum will depend on the presence of holes in the septum.

4.3.1 Key Diagnostic Points

4.3.1.1 Clinical Manifestations

1. Incomplete transverse vaginal septum: When the incomplete transverse septum is located in the upper vagina, it is usually asymptomatic and does not affect the sexual life and menstrual blood flow. However, if blood drainage is poor with intermittent flow, it can present as prolonged menstrual periods with continual spotting, and possibly leading to secondary infection. If the transverse septum is located at a lower position of the middle or lower part of the vagina, it would most likely affect the sexual life or cause sexual discomfort. Sometimes patient with transverse vaginal septum might manifest with primary infertility; or if pregnant, with obstructed labor and prolonged second stage of labor.
2. Complete transverse vaginal septum: Prepubertal patients are mostly asymptomatic; a few of them may have medical consultations due to abdominal pain or pelvic mass caused by vaginal and uterine blood accumulation; at and after adolescence, patients may present with primary amenorrhea, and with more blood retention in the lower abdomen causing cyclical pain or pelvic mass, sometimes they may also have urinary or bowel problems. Some patients have episodes of urinary retention and urinary tract infection. Untimely, treatment may result in reproductive tract infections and pelvic endometriosis.

4.3.1.2 Physical Examination

Gynecological examination revealed a short vagina, the top is a blind end or with small holes. The cervix could not be seen but above it, the uterus was palpable. If menstrual blood is retained, a mass can be palpable above the septum.

4.3.1.3 Imaging Examination

Examinations with ultrasonography, CT, or MRI can locate the transverse vaginal septum, reveal the degree of blood retention, and show the uterus and its adnexal findings. The combined applications of abdominal, perineal, vaginal, and rectal ultrasonography, CT, or MRI can provide a full preoperative evaluation of the reproductive tract anomalies and other malformations, especially the urinary tract anomaly. This helps to determine the surgical approach. Some scholars have proposed that intravenous pyelogram (IVP) should also be performed as a routine preoperative examination (Figs. 4.126 and 4.127).

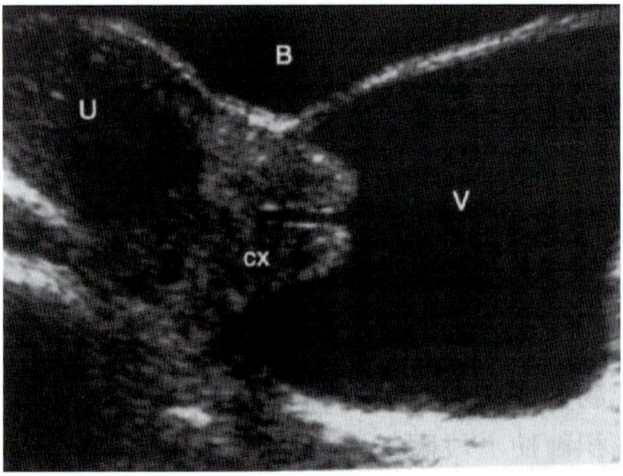

Fig. 4.126 Ultrasonography of retention of blood in the upper vagina

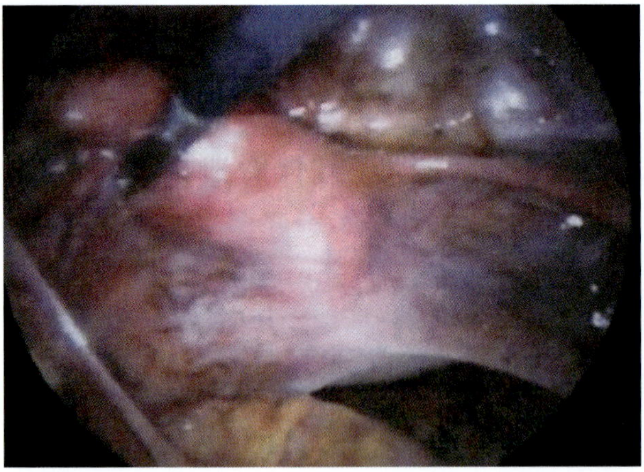

Fig. 4.127 Laparoscopy of the uterus and retention of blood in the upper vagina

4.3.2 Surgical Indications

1. When there is an accumulation of fluid or blood in the uterus, vagina, and even the fallopian tubes caused by the transverse vaginal septum
2. When sexual life is affected or is infertile
3. When it may prevent the descent of the presenting part in labor

4.3.3 Timing of Surgery

When a complete transverse vaginal septum is diagnosed after puberty and menarche, these patients should have surgical treatment carried out as soon as possible. For incomplete septum, if patients present with clinical symptoms before delivery or having infertility, surgical treatment is also recommended. If the transverse vaginal septum is diagnosed during pregnancy and is a thin septum, surgery can be performed to cut open the septum when the baby's presenting head presses upon the septum. After giving birth, septum resection should be then performed again as an elective surgery; if the septum is thick, cesarean section delivery should be chosen. In order to avoid injury to the bladder, urethra, and rectum, the timing of a safe surgery should be chosen when there is blood or fluid that accumulated above the septum causing some degree of distension in the upper part of the vagina.

4.3.4 Contraindications

1. When there is acute genital tract infection but not caused by the retention of blood or discharge, the infection should first be controlled with antibiotic before the surgery.
2. When there is no clear diagnosis of complex urogenital anomalies or accompanied cloacal malformation, no surgery should be performed.

4.3.5 Preoperative Preparation

1. Comprehensive assessment: A comprehensive assessment should include meticulous physical examination, ultrasonography, CT, MRI, and other relevant examinations. Other points of attention should be the age of the patient, history of pregnancy or infertility, other reproductive tract anomalies, etc. If the transverse septum is high in the vagina and close to the cervix, any associated cervical abnormality or cervical adhesion should be clearly defined. For incomplete transverse septum, a probe is used to define the thickness of the septum. Any associated local infection should be treated before the operation.
2. Adequate preoperative preparation: Preoperative preparation should include vulval skin cleaning, enema, and fasting 6 h before the surgery.
3. Preoperative counseling and explanation of the surgery: Preoperative examination and assessment should give a comprehensive understanding of the patient's condition before surgery. Through preoperative discussion, operative approach and possibility of any potential injury and accident are evaluated. Proper counseling is done by communicating the assessment with the patient and her family. As far as possible, the patient's fertility should be preserved.

4.3.6 Anesthesia

Local anesthesia or spinal anesthesia can be used depending on the location and thickness of the transverse vaginal septum and the general condition of the patient.

4.3.7 *Key Technical Points*

4.3.7.1 Transverse Vaginal Septum Excision

1. The patient should be in a lithotomy position. A large-pore needle is used to puncture a bulging area of the septum after careful palpation. When blood is sucked out from the puncture site, the septum is cut open by a pointed knife, on both sides of the punctured point, about 1 cm from left to right, so that the menstrual blood can be drained. The thickness of the transverse septum is evaluated. A vascular clamp is used to retract the incised transverse septum, sharply and bluntly upward till the upper and lower parts of the vagina are connected. The vagina is checked for any stenosis and the cervix is also examined for any anomaly. The transverse vaginal septum is excised as far as possible, by cutting off excessive septal tissue at about 0.5 ~ 1 cm from the base of the septum. The vaginal wound is sutured transversely and bleeding controlled with interrupted 2/0 absorbable sutures (Figs. 4.128 and 4.129).

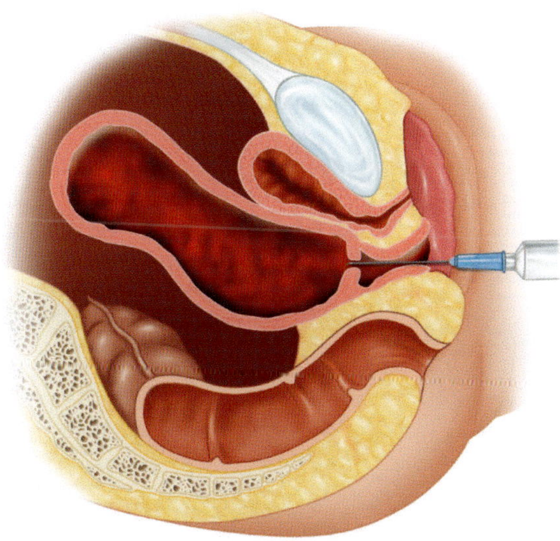

Fig. 4.128 Puncture with a long needle, blood clots aspirated to confirm the lesion

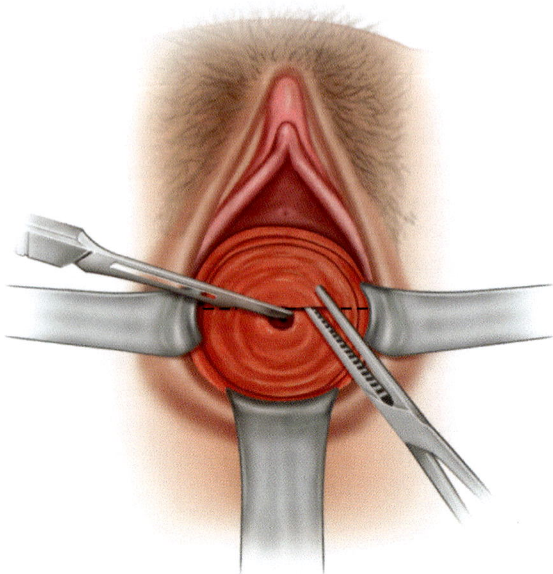

Fig. 4.129 Cut along the marked line

2. After cutting opened a transverse vaginal septum, a "pull-through" approach is employed; it is to identify the mucosal membrane on the upper part of the septum, then undermine and separate it from the septum. After the excision of the transverse septum, the mucosal membrane is pulled down and sutured to vaginal mucosal membrane below the cut septal wound to cover the raw area. Alternatively, another "push-through" approach is just the reverse by pushing up the mucosal membrane on the lower part of the septum and then suturing it with the upper vaginal mucosal membrane to cover the septal wound after the septum is excised. It had been reported that the push-through method has a lower risk of vaginal stenosis especially if the septum is thick with a wider septal wound after excision. Some scholars even suggested using a skin graft to bridge a thick septal wound (Fig. 4.130).

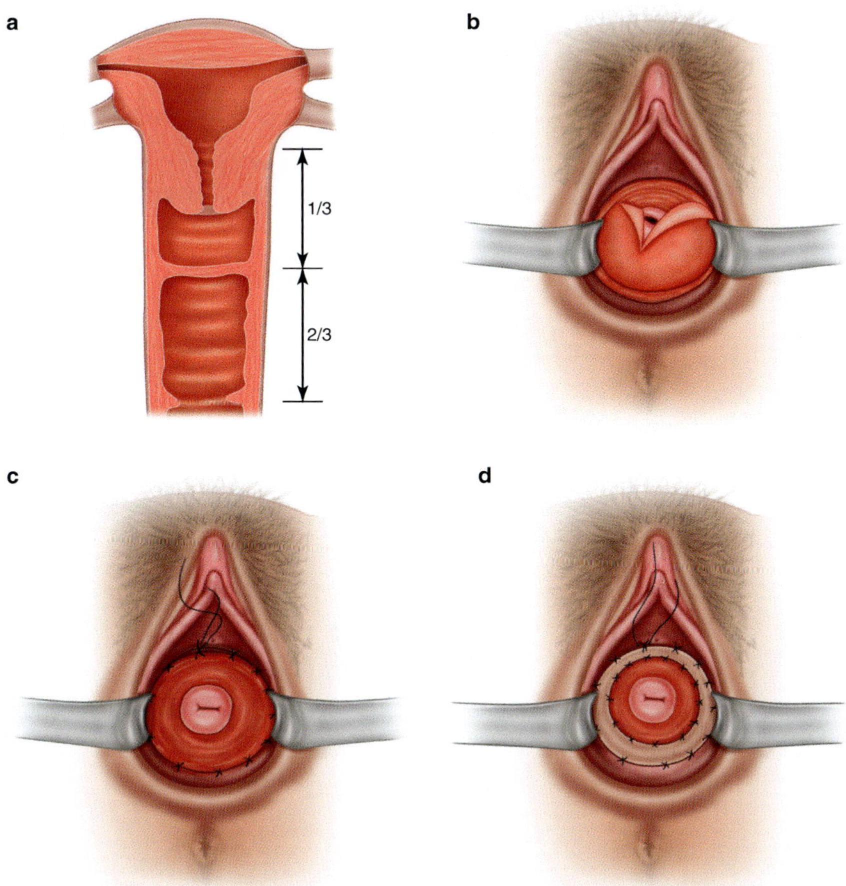

Fig. 4.130 Key points on the excision of a transverse vaginal septum. (a) A transverse vaginal septum; (b) cutting open the septum, expose the cervix; (c) suturing of the upper and lower edges of the mucosal membrane to cover the septal wound; (d) alternatively, skin flap is sutured in place to cover the septal wound surface of the excised transverse septum

3. If the transverse vaginal septum is diagnosed at delivery, it is wise to wait till the presenting part is pressing against the septum. The transverse septum can be cut in an "X" shape and removed after the baby is delivered (Fig. 4.131).

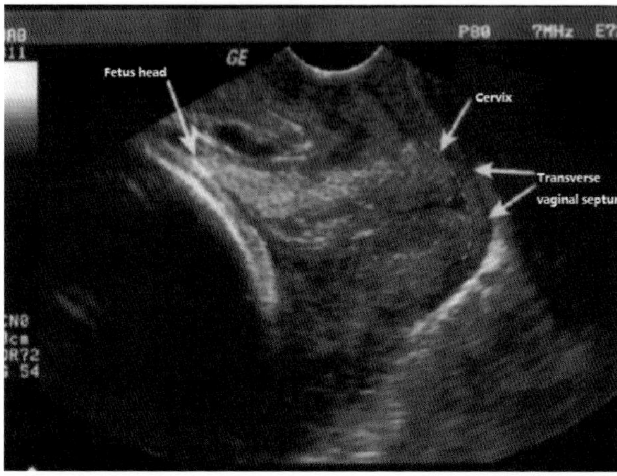

Fig. 4.131 Ultrasound scan finding of a transverse vaginal septum during pregnancy

Grunberger
"Z" plastic surgery (Grunberger surgical correction) (Fig. 4.132).

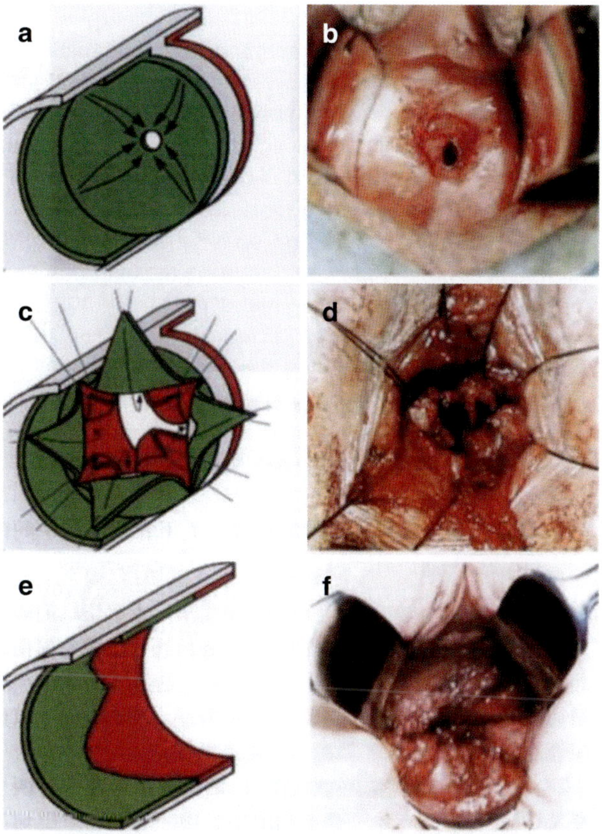

Fig. 4.132 Key points of "Z" plastic surgery. (**a**, **b**) Cut the outer membrane; (**c**, **d**) off the outer membrane, displace an angle of 45-degree, cut intima; (**e**, **f**) "Z" character formed

4.3.7.2 Technical Points of "Z" Plastic Surgery

1. The transverse vaginal septum is generally composed of three layers: the upper and lower mucosal membrane layers and the middle connective tissue layer. Saline water is injected into the middle layer of the septum to form a cushion to separate the upper and lower mucosal membranes. At the transverse vaginal septum, two sloping "X"-shaped incisions are made. Four triangular flaps of vaginal mucosal membrane are separated by sharp and blunt cutting. The slopping "X" triangular flaps will have a wide base which helps to avoid possible injury to the bladder and the rectum when the septum is excised. According to the pore size at the transverse septum, the connective tissue between the mucosal membranes should be removed completely. The top ends of the eight triangular mucosal flaps are marked with sutures (Fig. 4.132). During the operation, a Foley catheter can be inserted to the bladder in front and a rectal examination is performed behind to serve as position indictors to avoid injury to the urethra and rectum, respectively.
2. After two X incisions are made as above, the upper and lower vaginal mucosal membranes form a total of eight triangular vaginal flaps. These flaps should rotate at an angle of 45° to cross each other. It is important to avoid injury to the bladder and the rectum during these procedures. To facilitate the incision and dissection of the upper mucosal membrane of the septum, a balloon catheter can be inserted into a pore of the vaginal septum. A continuous traction is used at the end of the catheter to pull down and expand the septum, so as to simplify the procedure and avoid injury to the surrounding organs.
3. Before suturing the vaginal mucosal flaps, all the middle layer of connective tissues are excised and removed. The edges of the upper and lower vaginal mucosal flaps are trimmed nicely and made loose enough for anastomosis. The free edges of the upper and lower mucosal flaps are sutured in Z shape, i.e., the apex of a flap is sutured to the base of the intersection of two other flaps, so that the flaps are face to face. Absorbable sutures should be used and with interrupted single layer sutures. In this suturing approach, the flaps from two sides of the septum can naturally lengthen the vagina by 0.5 ~ 1 cm.

4.3.8 Postoperative Management

After operation, a vaginal mold is used and changed regularly until complete healing of the vaginal epithelium. This generally takes 6–8 weeks. Then a regular sex life can resume. If there is no expected sex, the mold should be used regularly for 6–24 months in order to reduce the incidence of postoperative vaginal stenosis. A rigid but hollow mold is more suitable and recommended.

4.4 Longitudinal Vaginal Septum

Xue Xiang

Longitudinal vaginal septum (Fig. 4.133) is due to developmental abnormalities of the lower end of the paramesonephric ducts. When the two ducts joined, the septum in between did not disappear (forming a complete longitudinal vaginal septum) or did not completely disappear (forming an incomplete longitudinal vaginal septum). For complete longitudinal vaginal septum (Fig. 4.134), the septum is generally attached to the anterior and the posterior wall of the vagina in the midline longitudinally, with equal-sized vaginas on both sides; if the septum does not lie in the midline, but deviated toward one side, then one vagina will be larger and the other smaller. Incomplete longitudinal vaginal septum is where the septum is not completely separating the vagina, usually only at the lower section, while vaginas in the upper section are connected.

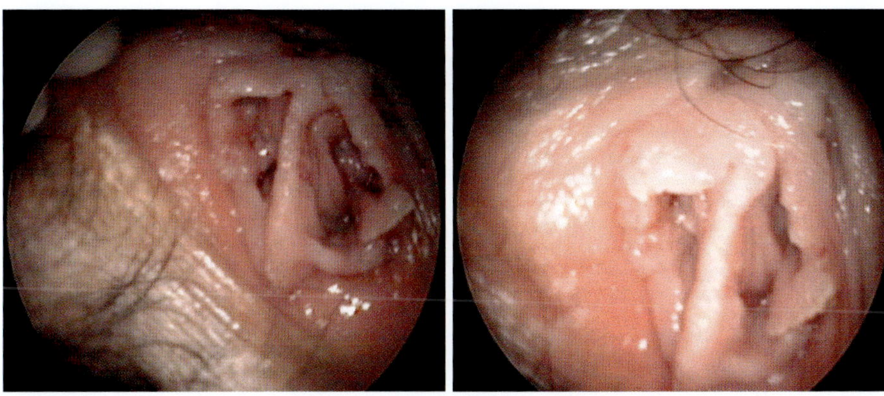

Fig. 4.133 Vaginal septum: hysteroscopic views of the vaginal openings

Longitudinal vaginal septum is sometimes associated with other reproductive tract anomalies, such as double uterus, double cervices, etc. (Figs. 4.135 and 4.136). When the vaginal septum is deviated to one side, it may have a vaginal atresia on that side, leading to menstrual blood retention. For complete longitudinal vaginal septum, sex may be within the vagina without ovulation and it may lead to infertility. If the vaginal anomaly is an incomplete longitudinal septum, with both upper vaginas being connected, there will not be any infertility problem. It is because no matter which side the intercourse takes place, semen can enter into the uterine cavity; thus, fertility is not affected.

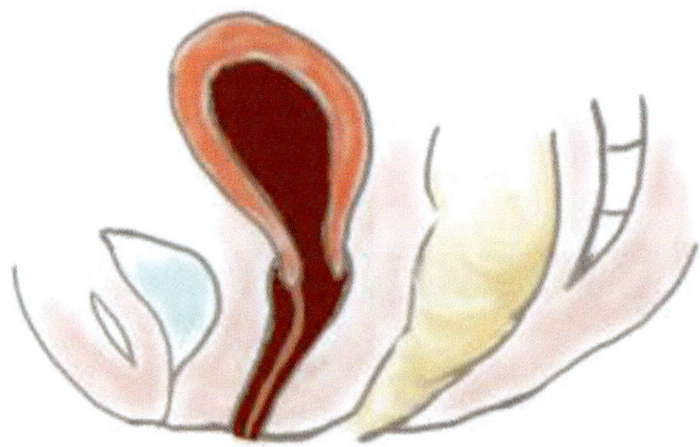

Fig. 4.134 A complete longitudinal septum

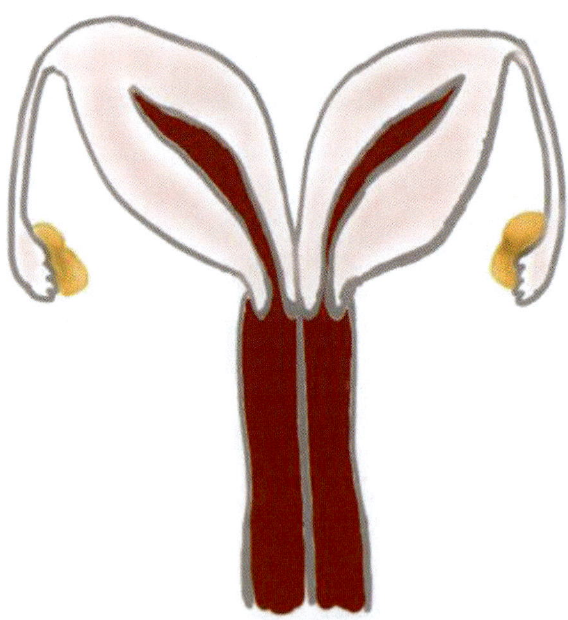

Fig. 4.135 A complete vaginal septum with double cervices and double uteri

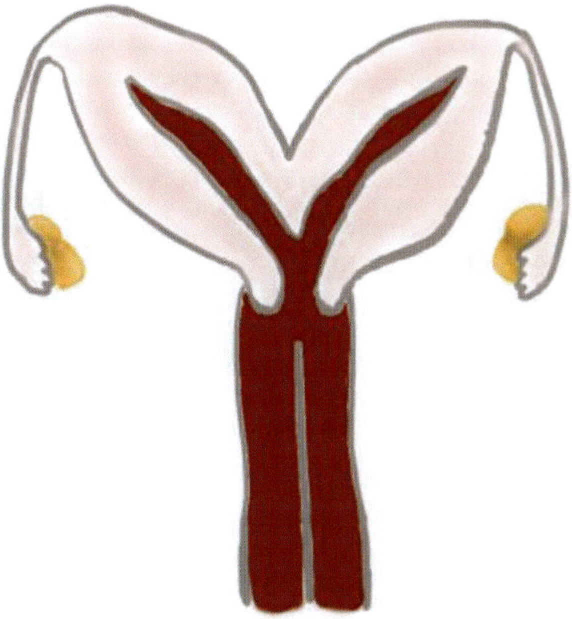

Fig. 4.136 An incomplete vaginal septum

4.4.1 Diagnosis

Longitudinal vaginal septum is mostly asymptomatic, and some are found only when there are sexual difficulties after marriage. Others may be confirmed as late as during delivery when progress of labor is slow. But for the following situations, the possibility of longitudinal vaginal septum should be considered.

1. During gynecological examination, a septum is found in the middle of the vagina.
2. There is difficulty in sexual intercourse.
3. During childbirth, the second stage of labor is slow or obstructed.
4. There is cyclical period pain if menstruation causes bleeding into the vagina and uterus in one side; ultrasound examination may reveal a cystic mass with blood clots.

4.4.2 Indications

Complete or incomplete longitudinal vaginal septum that affects sex life or impedes delivery.

4.4.3 Timing of Surgery

Surgery is usually scheduled at 3–7 days after the end of the menstruation. If it was not diagnosed before pregnancy, surgery should be performed immediately if it may affect vaginal delivery at the time of labor.

4.4.4 Contraindications

1. Patients with acute pelvic inflammatory disease or chronic pelvic inflammatory disease
2. Vaginal inflammation (such as trichomonas vaginitis, fungal vaginitis, bacterial vaginosis, etc.) and vulvitis
3. Other diseases that cannot tolerate surgery, e.g., coagulation defects

4.4.5 Preoperative Preparation

1. Gynecological examination should be carefully performed to define the conditions of the internal and external genitalia.
2. Routine investigations are performed for any leukorrhea so as to exclude vaginal infection like trichomonas vaginitis, fungal vaginitis, gonorrhea, etc.
3. Blood coagulation profile should be available to exclude abnormal blood test and coagulation defects.
4. Ultrasound examination for the uterus and adnexal mass is performed to look for other genital or urinary tract abnormalities.
5. Vulval skin preparation is carried out at the night before and the morning of surgery. Enema should also be given to prepare the bowel to prevent infection.
6. The vulva and vagina can be cleansed with 1:5000 potassium permanganate solution sitz bath three days and 0.05 % povidone-iodine prior to surgery.

4.4.6 Anesthesia

This surgery can be performed under local or spinal or general anesthesia.

4.4.7 Surgical Diagrams and Key Points of Surgical Techniques

1. Routine operative preparations are performed with vulval disinfection, strapping towels, and catheterization. The labia minora are sutured to the skin lateral to the labia majora on both sides so as to adequately expose the vaginal opening.

2. Gynecological examination is performed, using a finger to find out the relationship between the septum and the vaginal wall. A Sims speculum or other vaginal retractor can be used to open both sides of the vaginal wall in order to expose the longitudinal vaginal septum (Fig. 4.137).

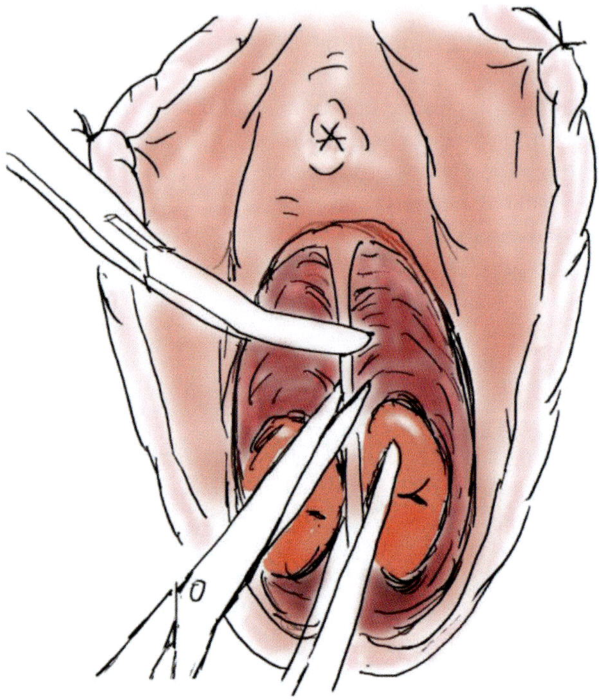

Fig. 4.137 The longitudinal vaginal septum is cut and removed alongside and in between two straight hemostats

3. Two straight hemostats are used to clamp the longitudinal vaginal septum, once or several times, at a distance of 0.5 cm from the anterior and posterior wall of the vagina, parallel to the vaginal wall, from outside to inside.
4. The vaginal septum is cut and removed, alongside and in between the two straight hemostats. Bleeding during the operation can be stopped with electric coagulation for hemostasis. If the septum is thin, cut off directly with an electric monopolar knife to reduce bleeding. During the cutting, it is important to avoid injury to the urethra and bladder in front and the rectum behind.

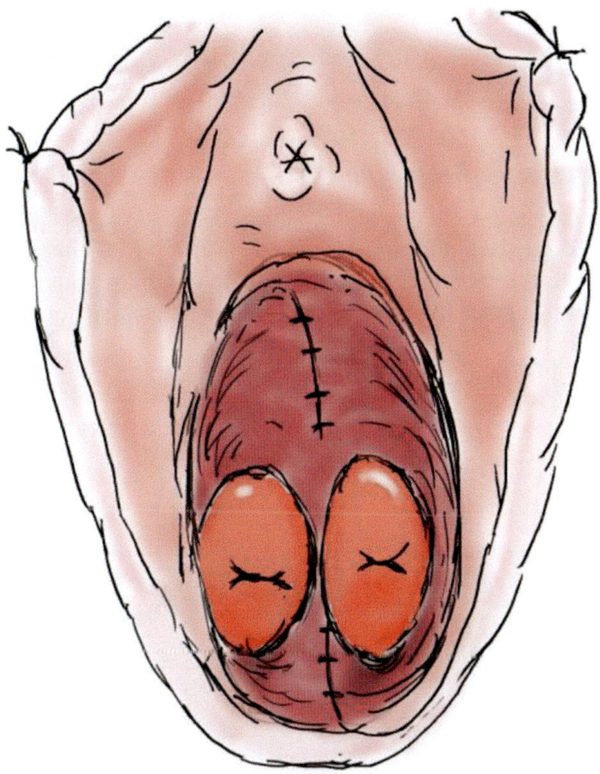

Fig. 4.138 The anterior and posterior septal wounds are sutured with continuously or interrupted sutures

5. Use No. 0 absorbable suture to suture from inside out continuously or interruptedly (Fig. 4.138). If the septum is very thin and there is no bleeding after excision, suturing may not be required.
6. If the vaginal septum is diagnosed during labor, it can be divided at its middle part. Sterile gauze can be inserted into the vagina temporarily to provide pressure for hemostasis. After the delivery of the fetus and placenta, the wound is inspected and excision of redundant septum can be completed. Suturing of wounds is then performed for hemostasis. Note if the vaginal septum has shrunk back or retracted after the initial cut. Care is taken such that the cutting should not be too close to the vaginal wall to avoid urethral, bladder, and bowel injury.
7. The vagina can be packed with Vaseline gauze to prevent adhesion after surgery.

4.4.8 Postoperative Management

1. The vaginal gauze packing should be removed at 12–24 h after operation.
2. Genital hygiene is maintained by cleaning with benzalkonium bromide (benzalkonium bromide) cotton ball to scrub the urethra and vaginal opening after toilet, to prevent infection.
3. Sexual intercourse should be prohibited for 30 days after operation.

4.5 Oblique Vaginal Septum Syndrome

Na Chen and Lan Zhu

4.5.1 *Diagnosis*

4.5.1.1 Definition

The oblique vaginal septum syndrome (OVSS) or Herlyn-Werner-Wunderlich syndrome (HWWS): It is a congenital genital anomaly which includes double uterus, double cervices, double vaginas with a complete or incomplete closed vagina. It is usually associated with an ipsilateral urinary tract malformation, commonly the absence of a kidney. There is an oblique septum covering one vagina, arising between the two cervices, running obliquely to the vaginal wall on one side. It covers the cervix, forming an isolated cavity between it and the cervix. In China, Bian Meilu in 1985 suggested the name of this malformation as oblique vaginal septum syndrome (OVSS); it is also known internationally as Herlyn-Werner-Wunderlich syndrome (HWWS) [1, 2].

4.5.1.2 The Origin

The pathogenesis of this condition remains unknown. According to some researchers, during the first 4 weeks of embryonic development, maldevelopment of the Wolffian duct and the ureteric bud on one side will be unable to guide the normal Mullerian duct on that side to fuse with the Mullerian duct on the contralateral side, which as a result will lead to the development of double sets of reproductive tract. An oblique septum is probably the blind end of a deviated Mullerian duct which at the 9th week of embryonic development extends incompletely and fails to fuse with the urogenital sinus. The end of it will form a blind tube resulting in the atresia of the cervix or vagina. The ureter bud maldevelopment will lead to the ipsilateral absence of kidney and ureter [2].

4.5.1.3 Types of Oblique Vaginal Septum

Type I – Oblique vaginal septum without holes: A vagina of one side is totally closed. The uterus behind the septum is totally separated to the outside and the other uterus. There is no connection between the two uteri and two vaginas. Retention of blood occurs in the cervix and uterus behind the septum. It is usually associated with an ipsilateral renal agenesis.

Type II – Oblique vaginal septum with holes: A vagina in one side is not totally closed. There is a hole of few mm in diameter in the septum. The uterus behind the septum is totally separated from the other uterus. Menstrual flow will go through the hole in the septum, but the flow is not smooth. It is also associated with an ipsilateral renal agenesis.

Type III – Oblique vaginal septum without holes but associated with a cervical fistula: A vagina in one side is totally closed, but there is a fistula between both cervices or between a cervix and the uterine cavity on the other side. The menstrual blood from the uterus behind the septum will go through the fistula and out from the other cervix, but the flow is not smooth. An ipsilateral renal agenesis is usually associated with it (Fig. 4.139).

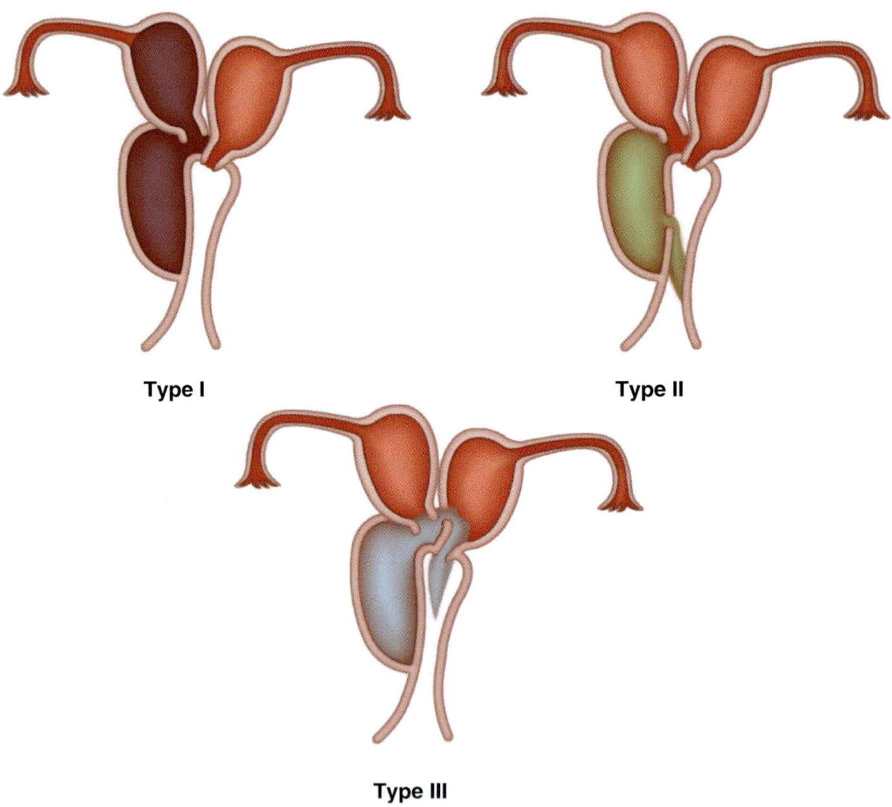

Fig. 4.139 Types of oblique vaginal septum syndrome

4.5.1.4 Clinical Manifestations

Clinical presentation depends on the types of oblique vaginal septum. In oblique septum type I, patients will complain of painful menarche and cystic mass. Patients with type II and type III oblique septum will present with prolonged menstrual spotting and purulent vaginal discharge.

4.5.2 Indications for Surgery

Surgery is indicated for patients who present with clinical symptoms and have the diagnosis confirmed. The septum should be removed as soon as diagnosed in types I, II, and III.

4.5.3 Contraindications

1. Other acute disease not under control
2. Significant local inflammation
3. Bleeding tendency
4. Uncertain diagnosis

4.5.4 Timing of Surgery

1. After an accurate diagnosis, the oblique septum should be removed early so as to relieve pain, to prevent infective complications, and to preserve fertility. If the treatment is delayed, complications like pelvic endometriosis, pelvic adhesions, and pelvic infection may lead to severe infection of the fallopian tube and the closed vagina.
2. Operation should be scheduled at the time of the menstruation, because the distending vaginal blood will help to mark the site of surgical puncture and make incision easier.

4.5.5 Preoperative Preparations

1. Acute infection or local inflammation if any should be under control with antibiotic.
2. Bowel preparation can be performed with laxative or enema to clean the bowel.

4.5.6 Anesthesia

Surgery can be performed with intravenous sedation, epidural, or general anesthesia.

4.5.7 Surgical Diagrams

Fig. 4.140.

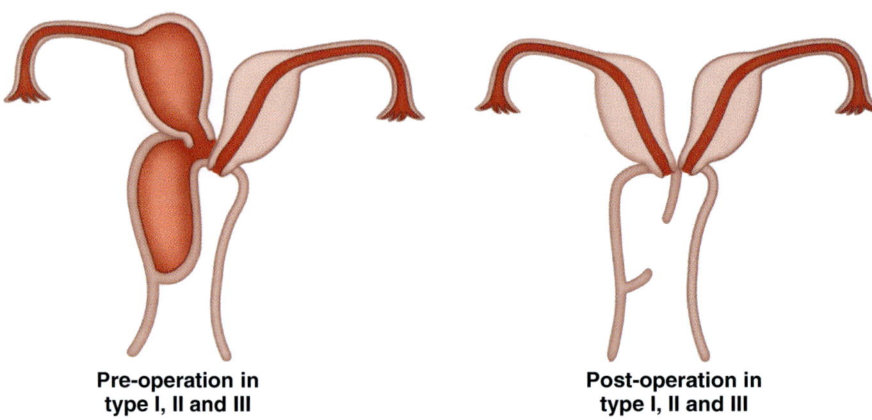

Fig. 4.140 Pre- and postoperation in types I, II, and III

4.5.8 Surgical Techniques

1. Total excision of oblique vaginal septum is the ideal operation for types I, II, and III. Just to cut open the septum should be avoided because the latter will lead to adhesive reclosure of the cut-opened septum.
2. At the time of operation, puncture should be performed either through the hole in the septum or at the most bulging part of the cystic mass. A successful aspiration of any old blood or pus will confirm the accurate position for incision.
3. It is important to have adequate excision of the oblique vaginal septum. After puncture, the oblique vaginal septum is cut open longitudinally up to the pouch of Douglas at the top and the lower part of the distended cyst at the vagina. Any excessive septum should be removed to allow smooth menstrual flow.
4. The key point is to avoid readhesive closure of the incised septal opening. After adequately exposing the cervix, the raw septum wound can be sutured with interrupted absorbable suture. The vagina should be packed with antiseptic gauze to provide pressure hemostasis and to prevent readhesion. The gauze is removed 48–72 h later.
5. In principle, it is not advisable to perform an abdominal hysterectomy to remove the affected uterus, because keeping the uterus may improve the ability to conceive.
6. Some authors recommended the use of hysteroscopic resection of the oblique septum and performed cleansing. This offers good result and does not damage the hymen [3].
7. Some have suggested laparoscopy should be performed for patients with oblique vaginal septum, who inevitably will develop blood reflux. Especially for teenagers, early diagnosis of endometriosis can prevent further distortion of the normal anatomy and loss of fertility [4].
8. For patients with types I, II, and III, some authors recommended combined laparoscopic and hysteroscopic surgery to diagnose and treat this condition. Laparoscopic hysterectomy can be performed to remove the underdeveloped uterus, while hysteroscopy can excise the oblique septum. But this combined surgical approach remains to be popularized.
9. Once the oblique vaginal septum has been surgically removed, the patient will have the same fertility potential as other normal women. For patients with types I, II, and III, their uteri can have normal pregnancy and delivery. However, a small number of patients may have miscarriage, retarded fetal growth, and ectopic pregnancy [1].

References

1. Lan Zhu, Na Chen, et al. New classification of Herlyn-Werner-Wunderlich Syndrome. Chin Med J. 2015;128(24):222–5.
2. Burgis J. Obstructive Müllerian anomalies: case report, diagnosis, and management. Am J Obstet Gynecol. 2001;185:338–44.

3. Xu B, Xue M, Xu D. Hysteroscopic management of an oblique vaginal septum in a virgin girl with a rare variant of Herlyn-Werner-Wunderlich syndrome. J Minim Invasive Gynecol. 2015;22(1):7.
4. Hur JY, Shin JH, Lee JK, Oh MJ, Saw HS, Park YK, et al. Septate uterus with double cervices, unilaterally obstructed vaginal septum, and ipsilateral renal agenesis: a rare combination of Müllerian and Wolffian anomalies complicated by severe endometriosis in an adolescent. J Minim Invasive Gynecol. 2007;14:128–31.

Suggested Reading

Beyth Y, Klein Z, Weinstein S, et al. Thick transverse vaginal septum: expectant management followed by surgery. J Pediatr Adolesc Gynecol. 2004;17(6):379–81.

Blanton EN, Rouse DJ. Trial of labor in women with transverse vaginal septa. Obstet Gynecol. 2003;101(5):1110–2.

Cetinkaya K, Kumtepe Y. Perforated transverse vaginal septum: a rare case of Mullerian duct anomaly presenting only primary infertility. Fertil Steril. 2008;90(5):2005e.11–13.

Decherney AH. Current obstetrics and gynecology diseases diagnosis and treatment. 1998. p. 77–89.

Fujimoto VY, Miller JH, Klein NA, et al. Congenital cervical atresia: report of seven cases and review of the literature. Am J Obstet Gynecol. 1997;177:1419–25.

Grund D, Köhler C, Krauel H, Schneider A. A new approach to preserve fertility by using a coated nitinol stent in a patient with recurrent cervical stenosis. Fertil Steril. 2007;88(3):763–4.

Jinhua L, Jinghe L, Lijuan L, et al. Vagina atresia: a clinical analysis of 16 cases. Chin J Obstetr Gynecol. 2002;37(4):217–9.

Joki-Erkkilä MM, Heinonen PK. Presenting and long-term clinical implications and fecundity in females with obstructing vaginal malformations. Pediatr Adolesc Gynecol. 2003;16(5): 307–12.

Lacy J, Correll GR, Walmer DK, et al. Simple vaginal mold for use in the postoperative care of patients with a transverse vaginal septum. Fertil Steril. 2007;87(5):1225–6.

Lang Jinghe. Gynecology surgical notes, vol 2. China Science and Technology Press; 2004. p. 45–9.

Liu Xinmin. Gynecologic surgery study, 3rd edn. People's Medical Publishing House; 2003; p. 558–60.

Nazir Z, Rizvi RM, Qureshi RN, et al. Congenital vaginal obstructions: varied presentation and outcome. Pediatr Surg Int. 2006;22(9):749–53.

Polasek PM, Erickson LD, Stanhope CR. Transverse vaginal septum associated with tubal atresia. Mayo Clin Proc. 1995;70(10):965–8.

Quint EH, McCarthy JD, Smith YR. Vaginal surgery for congenital anomalies. Clin Obstet Gynecol. 2010;53(1):115–24.

Rana A, Manandhar B, Amatya A, et al. Mucocolpos due to complete transverse septum in middle third of vagina in a 17-year-old girl. J Obstet Gynaecol Res. 2002;28(2):86–8.

Ribeiro SC, Yamakami LY, Tormena RA. Septate uterus with cervical duplication and longitudinal vaginal septum. Rev Assoc Med Bras. 2010;56(2):254–6.

Roberts CP, Rock JA. Surgical methods in the treatment of congenital anomalies of the uterine cervix. Curr Opin Obstet Gynecol. 2011;23(4):251–7. Review.

Simpson JL. Anomalies of internal ducts. In: Simpson JL, editor. Disorders of sexual differentiation: etiology and clinical delineation. San Diego: Academic; 1976. p. 341–59.

Wang J, Ezzat W, Davidson M. Transverse vaginal septum. A case report. J Reprod Med. 1995;40(2):163–6.

Wierrani F, Bodner K, Spängler B, et al. "Z"-plasty of the transverse vaginal septum using Garcia's procedure and the Grünberger modification. Fertil Steril. 2003;79(3):608–12.

Chapter 5
Abnormal Uterine Development

Sumin Wang, Feng Xu, Limin Feng, and Xue Xiang

5.1 Rudimentary Horn

Sumin Wang

A rudimentary horn of the uterus is caused by a defective fusion of the paramesonephric ducts. One paramesonephric duct usually develops normally, while the contralateral one can develop into various degrees of rudimentary horns [1]. The incidence is about 0.1 % [2]. Patients usually consult doctors because of infertility, recurrent miscarriage, or chronic pelvic pain [3]. The incidences of rudimentary horn in patients with a medical history of miscarriage, infertility, and recurrent miscarriage are 0.5, 0.5, and 3.1 % [1].

5.1.1 Diagnosis

A rudimentary horn, with or without its uterine cavity, is usually not connected with the other unicornuate uterine cavity. The rudimentary horn may be free or may be connected to the unicornuate uterus by a fibrous cord. It is commonly located at the

S. Wang (✉) • F. Xu
Department of Obstetrics and Gynecology, Nanjing Maternity and Infant Hospital of Nanjing Medical University, Nanjing, Jiangsu, P. R. China
e-mail: 115657929@qq.com, xfnjcn@hotmail.com

L. Feng
Department of Gynaecology, Beijing Tiantan Hospital, The Capital University of Medical Sciences, Beijing 100050, China

X. Xiang
Department of Gynaecology & Obstetrics, The Second Affiliated Hospital, Medical School of Xi'an Jiaotong University, Xi'an, China

© Springer Science+Business Media Dordrecht 2015
L. Zhu et al. (eds.), *Atlas of Surgical Correction of Female Genital Malformation*,
DOI 10.1007/978-94-017-7246-4_5

middle or lower part of the developed unicornuate uterus. Occasionally, they are found and located at the fundal part of the uterus. It has a normal fallopian tube, ovary, and ligament development. According to Buttram and Gibbons' classification as well as AFS classification of uterine malformations in 1979, type II is a unicornuate uterus. This type of uterine anomaly can be divided into four types according to the development of the undeveloped uterus and its relationship with the developed uterus:

IIA: There is a developed unicornuate uterus on one side and the other one is a rudimentary horn.

- Ia: The rudimentary horn is abnormally developed with a uterine cavity but without a cervix. It can connect with the unicornuate uterus.
- Ib: The rudimentary horn is abnormally developed with a uterine cavity but without a cervix, and it is not connected with the unicornuate uterus.
- Ic: The rudimentary horn is a primordial uterus which is abnormally developed. It has no uterine entity, has no cervix, and is connected to the unicornuate uterus by a bundle of fibrous cords.

IIB: The unicornuate uterus is well developed with a fallopian tube, an ovary, and the round ligament, but there is no uterus on the other side as it is completely underdeveloped.

The European Society of Human Reproduction and Embryology (ESHRE) and the European Society for Gynaecological Endoscopy (ESGE) in June 2013 formed the "CONgenital UTerine Anomalies (CONUTA)" working group which based on the embryonic origin and anatomy released a new classification of congenital anomalies of the female reproductive tract [4]. The classification divided the uterine anomalies into different main types, and these anomalies were further divided into different subtypes based on its severity and clinical significance. According to ESHRE/ESGE classification, both type U4 hemi-uterus and type U5 aplastic uterus have the presence of rudimentary horn anomalies. The differences of types U4 and U5 lie in the existence of a well-developed functional hemi-uterus. Due to the functional endometrial cavity in the rudimentary horn, it often leads to clinical manifestations of periodic abdominal pain, pelvic hematoma, and ectopic pregnancy, etc, many of which need surgical treatment, so depending on whether the rudimentary horn cavity is functional or not, further subtypes of U4 and U5 are classified.

Class U4 or hemi-uterus is defined as unilateral uterine development; the contralateral part could be either incompletely formed or absent. It is further divided into two subclasses depending on the presence or not of a functional rudimentary cavity:

1. U4a: Unicornuate (hemi-)uterus communicating with or not with contralateral functional rudimentary horn.
2. U4b: Unicornuate (hemi-)uterus without a functional rudimentary horn or no horn.

Class U5 or aplastic uterus incorporates all cases of uterine aplasia. There could be bi- or unilateral rudimentary horns with cavity, while in others, there could

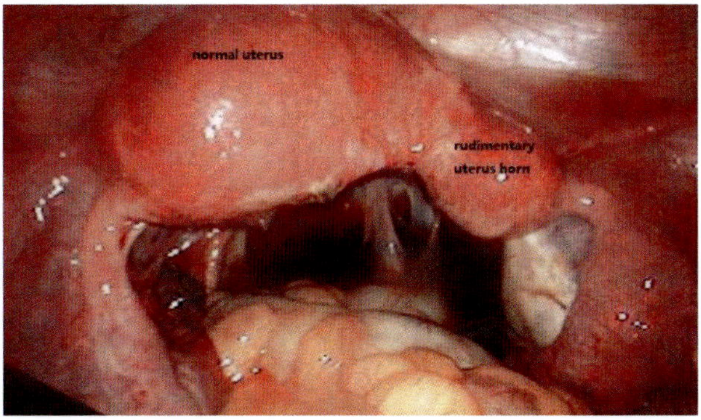

Fig. 5.1 A right rudimentary horn with a normal developed left uterus. There is pelvic endometriosis

be uterine remnants without cavity. Depending on the presence or not of a functional cavity in an existent rudimentary horn, class U5 is further divided into two subclasses:

1. U5a: Aplastic uterus with rudimentary (functional) cavity characterized by the presence of bi- or unilateral functional horn.
2. U5b: Aplastic uterus without rudimentary (functional) cavity characterized either by the presence of uterine remnants or by full uterine aplasia.

The clinical symptoms depend on the type of rudimentary horns. Periodic abdominal pain is the main reason for patients to seek medical consultation. Ruptured ectopic pregnancy is more dangerous in those with rudimentary functional horn, thus of great clinical importance. When a functional rudimentary horn communicates with a developed hemi-uterus, menstrual blood can be discharged; if not communicating or connected with only a fiber band or a very small communicating tube, menstrual blood cannot be discharged or will be poorly discharged. Patients with functional endometrium of the rudimentary horn can have cyclical periodic pain, blood in the uterine cavity, hematosalpinx, and pelvic endometriosis (Fig. 5.1). Type IIA-Ic or U5b rudimentary horn has only a primordial horn or uterine aplasia without functional endometrium. It is often easily misdiagnosed as a subserosal fibroid.

The key to ultrasound diagnosis of rudimentary horn and hemi-uterus is to display the uterine shape on the coronal plane and to identify whether there is asymmetrical uterine appearance. The fundus of the uterus appears narrow, with its endometrium deviating to one side like a lancet-shaped endometrial cavity. Further examination should be done to find the rudimentary horn. If a rudimentary horn is found, the presence of endometrium in the rudimentary horn cavity and its connection with the normal hemi-uterus should be defined. Depending on whether the rudimentary horn is functional or not, further subtypes are defined [3, 5]. A rudimentary horn without functional cavity or retained blood due to hemorrhage can easily be misdiagnosed as a uterine fibroid or degenerative fibroid, but 3D ultrasound however can display the uterine morphology for identification. Hysterosalpingography (HSG) is helpful in the diagnosis of rudimentary horn, with its typical banana sign. Here, the contrast

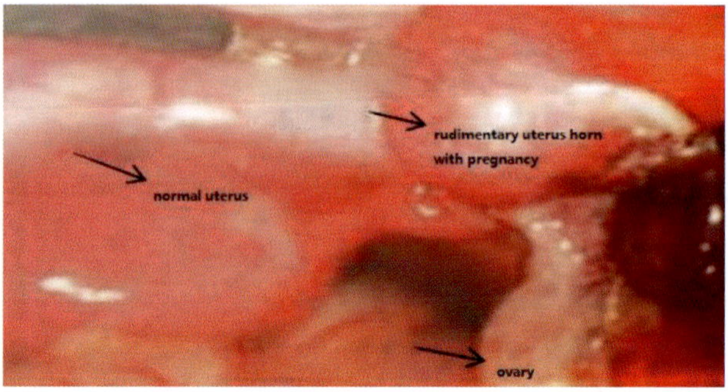

Fig. 5.2 Laparoscopic visualization of rudimentary horn pregnancy

medium enters further into the fallopian tube on one side. If the rudimentary horn and the developed hemi-uterus are connected, the contrast medium will be seen entering into the rudimentary horn. However, if hysterosalpingography does not show a rudimentary horn, diagnosis cannot be assumed because of a lack of connection between the rudimentary horn and the developed hemi-uterus [3]. MRI can clearly show whether the rudimentary horn has an endometrium or not and whether it is connected with the uterine cavity of the developed hemi-uterus; therefore, MRI can clearly diagnose the types of rudimentary horn [6]. CT angiography can also clearly reveal the blood supply of the rudimentary horn. However, ultrasound saline hysterosalpingogram and hysteroscopy examination remain the standard assessment and diagnostic method of uterine anomalies [7]. Those with obstructed menstrual flow should be alerted for possible pelvic endometriosis. Blood CA125 can help diagnose the coexistence of endometriosis.

In view of the common origin of the urinary system and the reproductive system during their embryonic development, patients who are suspected of having uterine malformation should undergo conventional ultrasound or MRI examinations to check for the status of the kidneys. This may, for example, be found on the same side as the rudimentary horn; there is an absence of an ipsilateral kidney, an ectopic kidney, a horseshoe kidney, or other cystic renal dysplasia, etc. Patients with type U5 aplastic uterus are often associated with other malformations, such as vaginal anomalies or MRHK syndrome [4].

A fertilized egg can embed in the rudimentary horn, grow, and develop into a rudimentary horn pregnancy (Fig. 5.2). There are four possible mechanisms of pregnancy:

1. Sperms from the uterine cavity of the developed uterus pass through a small communicating tube joining the rudimentary horn, then to its fallopian tube. Pregnancy in the rudimentary horn will occur after they fertilize the egg ovulated from the ovary on the side of the rudimentary horn. The fertilized egg then embeds in the uterine cavity of the rudimentary horn.
2. Sperms travel from the uterine cavity and out of the fallopian tube of the developed uterus, through the peritoneal cavity to the fallopian tube of the rudimentary horn. This will result in pregnancy after they fertilize the egg ovulated from the ovary. The fertilized egg subsequently embeds in the cavity of the rudimentary horn.

3. Sperms and eggs from the developed side travel through the peritoneal cavity to the fallopian tube of the rudimentary horn, resulting in pregnancy. The fertilized egg embeds in the cavity of the rudimentary horn.
4. The fertilized egg travels out from the fallopian tube of the developed side, via the peritoneal cavity to the fallopian tube of the rudimentary horn, and embeds and develops inside the rudimentary horn.

The survival rate of the fetus in rudimentary horn pregnancy is only 0–13 %. Rudimentary horn pregnancy is generally asymptomatic in the early stage. Fifty percent rudimentary horn pregnancy will rupture spontaneously, of which more than 80 % ruptures in rudimentary horn pregnancy occurred in midtrimester pregnancy, far later than ruptured tubal pregnancy.

At midtrimester pregnancy, because of the thin uterine wall of the undeveloped rudimentary horn, rupture typically occurs spontaneously, causing sudden onset of severe abdominal pain and hemorrhagic shock. This will endanger the life of the pregnant patient, with a mortality rate of 0.5–23 %.

When rudimentary horn communicates with the hemi-uterus, rudimentary horn pregnancy has similar symptoms as a tubal ectopic pregnancy, with a history of amenorrhea, abdominal pain, and vaginal bleeding. However, 80 % of rudimentary horn pregnancies occur in non-communicating rudimentary horns. The symptoms of these rudimentary horn pregnancies are similar to those in normal pregnancy without vaginal bleeding, but they will rupture at a later time.

Mostly at 12–26 weeks of pregnancy, they present with complete or incomplete uterine rupture, causing severe internal bleeding. When rudimentary horn pregnancy enlarges the horn, one should be aware of the risk of torsion of a rudimentary uterine horn pregnancy [8]. If the rudimentary horn has no functional uterine cavity, it will not result in rudimentary horn pregnancy; rarely, however, a tubal pregnancy on the side of rudimentary horn can still be possible.

The diagnostic criterion for rudimentary horn pregnancy is to use the round ligament as a guide. If the fetal sac is located medial to the round ligament attachment, it is a rudimentary horn pregnancy. If it is located lateral to the round ligament attachment, it is a tubal pregnancy. As a patient with rudimentary horn may have a normal vagina and cervix, but a small rudimentary horn, it is difficult to make a diagnosis based solely on bimanual pelvic examination before pregnancy. Patients with a history of infertility, premature labor, and spontaneous miscarriage should undergo both ultrasound scan and MRI to exclude uterine anomalies and ectopic uterine pregnancy. Three-dimensional ultrasound on rudimentary uterine pregnancy is a particularly effective diagnostic tool. The key points of 3D ultrasound diagnosis are the absence of a cervix in the pregnant uterus and presence of another nonpregnant uterus. Then the application of 3D imaging can observe the morphology of the hemi-uterus cavity, confirming the absence of a pregnancy sac. The endometrium is like a lancet pointing to one side of its uterine horn. In the lower end of the uterus, there is a tissue mass echo (i.e., rudimentary uterine horn); visible within it is a pregnancy sac or embryo. But the pregnancy sac and cervix are not connected. These findings can be diagnosed as rudimentary horn pregnancy [9, 10].

In suspected cases, either MRI or combined laparoscopy and hysteroscopy can be performed to confirm the diagnosis.

5.1.2 Indications

1. Rupture of rudimentary horn pregnancy is an acute abdominal condition requiring emergency surgery [10, 11].
2. For patients with abdominal pain, particularly those with cyclical abdominal pain, in order to avoid secondary dysmenorrhea, endometriosis, and rudimentary horn pregnancy, it is recommended that the rudimentary horn should be prophylactically removed [12, 13].
3. For patients with asymptomatic rudimentary horn, if ultrasound or MRI confirms that there is uterine endometrium, the rudimentary horn should be prophylactically removed [14].
4. Whether to remove a rudimentary horn with nonfunctional endometrium is in dispute. Removal of this rudimentary horn does not improve pregnancy outcome.

5.1.3 Timing of Surgery

Depending on the different timing and circumstances when a rudimentary horn is diagnosed, different surgical approaches could be chosen.

For nonpregnancy, it will be practical to perform the resection of rudimentary horn and ipsilateral salpingectomy while the ipsilateral ovary can be preserved. The ipsilateral round ligament and ovary should be suspended over the side of the developed uterus. The location should be opposite to the contralateral round ligament, tube, and ovary of the developed uterus. This is to prevent any torsion of the uterus. With regard to fertility considerations, in patients with abnormalities or absence of the contralateral fallopian tube, there are reports of surgical transplantation of fallopian tube together with its associated uterine horn. For patients with coexistent endometriosis, appropriate surgical treatment should be performed depending on the location of the endometriosis. Patients without fertility issue, radical excision of endometriosis can be performed.

Rupture of the rudimentary horn pregnancy, once diagnosed, should have surgical treatment performed as soon as possible. Patients with acute abdomen and internal bleeding should preferably be explored by laparotomy; if there are no signs of acute internal bleeding or there are stable vital signs, then laparoscopy is acceptable. During early and midtrimester pregnancy, resection of a rudimentary horn and ipsilateral tubal ligation or resection are appropriate to prevent future recurrence of ectopic pregnancy on the side of the rudimentary horn. But the ovary should be preserved and be suspended over the side of the developed uterus. When the pregnancy has reached full term and for those with live births, cesarean section should be performed to save the fetus; the rudimentary horn and ipsilateral fallopian tube should be removed at the same time. Patients without further reproductive demands may consider hysterectomy and bilateral salpingectomy.

5.1.4 Contraindications

Type II A-1c or U5b rudimentary horn is a primordial uterus, while the aplastic uterus has no uterine body and cavity. Whether it is necessary to remove a rudimentary horn with no functional endometrium is still under debate. Also the removal of this type of rudimentary horn does not improve pregnancy outcome.

5.1.5 Preoperative Preparation

1. Investigation with IVU (intravenous urogram) or MRI is necessary to determine if there is any urinary tract abnormality. If confirmed, a urologist should be consulted for planning a joint operation to avoid multiple surgeries on the same patient. Also, the course and location of the ureters can be determined.
2. For nonpregnancy surgery, CT angiography may help to determine the blood supply of the rudimentary horn and select the most suitable surgical procedure.
3. For patients with dysmenorrhea, serum CA125 can be taken to determine the presence of endometriosis.
4. Preoperative preparations are as for other routine gynecological surgery.
5. In case of rupture of rudimentary horn pregnancy, blood should be reserved for blood transfusion.

5.1.6 Anesthesia

The patient is placed in a lithotomy position, and general anesthesia with tracheal intubation is performed.

5.1.7 Laparoscopic Resection of Rudimentary Horn

Key surgical techniques [14, 15]:

1. The round ligament is ligated and cut on the side of the rudimentary horn. The ipsilateral fallopian tube is removed, but the ovary is preserved. When no ovary is found in the pelvis, the descending path of the ovarian development should be

explored. Intraoperative ultrasound examination can be used when it is necessary. Keeping detailed records of the ovarian finding is to benefit the patient to seek assisted reproductive technology (ART) for pregnancy.

2. The ovarian uterine ligament is ligated and cut on the side of the rudimentary horn.
3. The uterine artery of the rudimentary horn is identified, cut, and controlled by using bipolar coagulation, ultrasonic scalpel, suture, etc. When the uterine artery is to be cut, the position of the ureter must be identified because the vascular supply to the rudimentary horn is directly from the ipsilateral uterine artery, and the ureter may also have shifted higher on the same side.
4. During removal of the rudimentary horn, care should be taken to avoid removal of too much myometrium of the developed uterus. The hemostasis of the cut raw surface can be controlled by electric coagulation or suture.
5. After removal of the rudimentary horn, the ipsilateral ovary and round ligament are sutured and suspended onto the side of the developed uterus. The location should be chosen so as to be opposite to the contralateral accessories and round ligament of the developed uterus. This helps to prevent the possibility of torsion of a pregnant uterus in the future.
6. The resected rudimentary horn can be removed via the pouch of Douglas of the vagina or by an electric morcellator via a trocar in the abdominal wall. Figure 5.3 shows examples of specimens of removed rudimentary uterine horn and ipsilateral fallopian tube.
7. At the time of the operation, if the rudimentary horn is found to be distended with retained blood, it can be cut opened to drain the blood; if infection is suspected, blood sample should be taken for bacterial culture and broad-spectrum antibiotics should be given. If careful exploration revealed infection-induced fistula formation between the rudimentary horn and vagina, either laparotomy or laparoscopy combined with vaginal surgery is required to surgically close the fistula [16].
8. For a patient with coexisting endometriosis, appropriate surgical treatment should be performed according to location of the endometriosis.

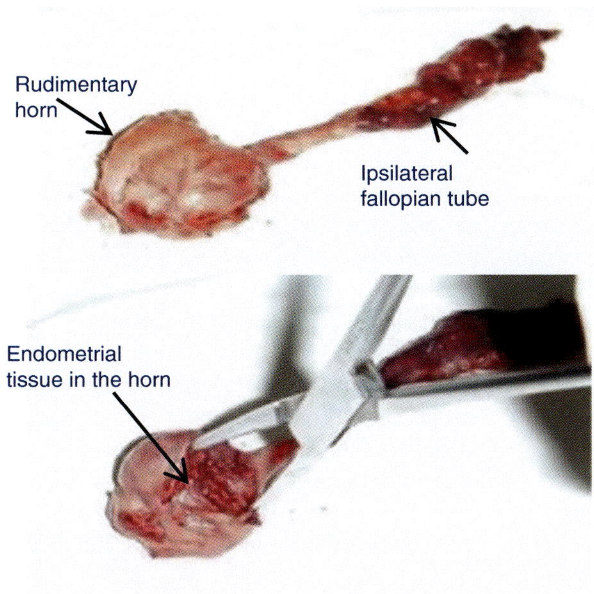

Fig. 5.3 Specimens of rudimentary horn and ipsilateral fallopian tube removed through the pouch of Douglas from the vagina

5.2 T-Shaped Uterus

Sumin Wang and Feng Xu

Diethylstilbestrol (DES) is a synthetic estrogen which can increase the production of steroid hormone from the placenta during pregnancy, thus reducing the incidence of miscarriages and premature births. It had been widely used from 1948 to 1971 for the treatment for recurrent miscarriages. It was until the relationship of vaginal clear cell carcinoma and the effects of fetal in utero exposure to DES were discovered that its use was then stopped [17]. Early in utero exposure to diethylstilbestrol during pregnancy caused vaginal clear cell carcinoma in only 0.1 % of these patients, while the incidence of the reproductive tract abnormalities occurred in 35–69 % with DES exposure in utero. The uterine abnormality was dose related, and uterine hypoplasia and T-shaped uterine cavity were the most common uterine anomalies. Female fetuses with exposure to DES in utero presented in their adult life with problems of infertility, ectopic pregnancy, spontaneous abortion, and premature delivery [18]. Intrauterine adhesions at lower end of the uterine cavity can also cause uterine narrowing, forming a T-shaped uterine cavity [19].

5.2.1 Diagnosis

According to Buttram and Gibbons (1979) and the American Fertility Society (1988) classification of uterine anomalies, class VII uterine anomalies are related to exposure to DES in utero [20, 21] (Fig. 5.4):

The European Society of Human Reproduction and Embryology (ESHRE) and the European Association of Gynecologic Endoscopy (ESGE) in June 2013 had established a working group under the name of CONUTA (CONgenital UTerine Anomalies) and presented a new consensus ESHRE/ESGE classification system [22]. Type U1 uterine cavity abnormalities (dysmorphic uterus) showed the normal uterine outline but with an abnormal shape of the uterine cavity, usually of small uterine volume. Class 1 is further subdivided into three categories (Fig. 5.5): U1a or T-shaped uterus, characterized by a narrow uterine cavity due to the lateral thickening of the uterine side wall, with a correlation 2/3 uterine corpus and 1/3 cervix; type U1b or uterus infantilis is characterized by a narrow uterine cavity without lateral wall thickening and an inverse correlation of 1/3 uterine body and 2/3 cervix; and type U1c or others, which is added to include all minor uterine cavity abnormalities, such as those with an inner indentation at the fundal midline level of <50 % of the uterine wall thickness. This aims to facilitate groups who want to study patients with minor abnormalities and to clearly differentiate them from patients with septate uterus.

Patients with exposure to DES in utero have reduced fertility and higher incidence of ectopic pregnancy, spontaneous abortion, and premature birth rate than normal women [18, 23]. Their full-term delivery rate in their first pregnancy was 64.1 %, compared to the 84.5 % in those without DES in utero exposure. Further research found that the incidence rates for spontaneous abortion, premature birth, and ectopic pregnancy of women exposed to DES in utero were 19.2 %, 11.5 %, and 4.2 %, respectively, in their first pregnancy, while for those without DES exposure were 10.3 %, 4.1 %, and 0.77 %. Therefore, when the reproductive history of those exposed to DES in utero was analyzed, these patients were more prone to premature birth, early trimester and midtrimester miscarriages, ectopic pregnancy, and so on.

Vaginal ultrasonography can be difficult in detecting DES-related uterine anomalies, while HSG examination is the preferred examination for DES-related uterine anomalies (Fig. 5.6); HSG can define the characteristic T-shaped uterine cavity, with narrow uterine cavity and irregular uterine edge. When combined with a history of exposure to DES in utero, this would lead to a further MRI examination if available to confirm the diagnosis. MRI examination can show the main features of the uterine anomalies caused by DES exposure such as the narrow and irregular uterine cavity, a shorter horizontal uterine segment, and a narrow vertical uterine segment marked by a narrowed band. This band is due to the local thickening of the uterine muscle tissue on both sides. These imaging studies showed the characteristic T-shaped uterine cavity; MRI also can find abnormal cervical development with narrow irregular cervical canal and so on. However, MRI would be difficult to find any tubal abnormality, and it may need saline hydrosonography to assist its diagnosis [24]. HSG and MRI showed a T-shaped uterine cavity, but they still cannot distinguish between various subtypes of T-shaped uterus. Further investigations with hysteroscopy and cervical and endometrial biopsies may be required to confirm the differential diagnosis [25].

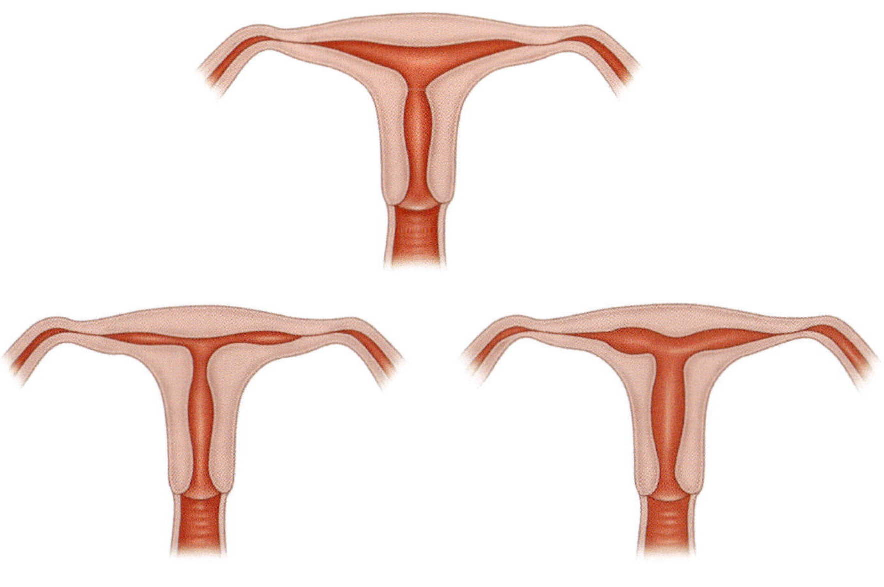

Fig. 5.4 American Fertility Society classification of uterine anomalies – class VII diagrams (Emans SJ, Laufer MR, Goldstein DP. *Pediatric and adolescent gynecology*. 5th ed. Philadelphia: Lippincott Williams & Wilkins Publishing Company; 2005)

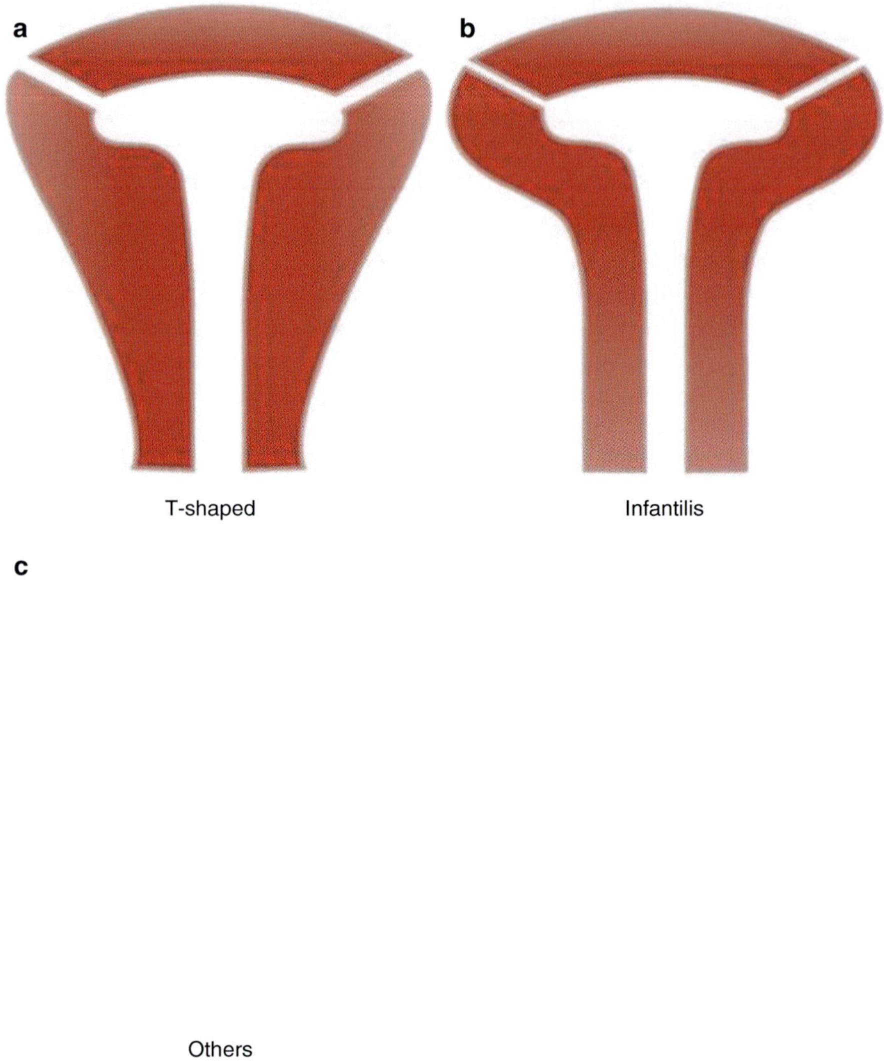

Fig. 5.5 ESHRE/ESGE classification of uterine anomalies of type U1 (Grimbizis et al. [4]). Type U1 is further subdivided into three categories U1a or T-shaped uterus, U1b or uterus infantilis and Type U1c or others. The last one is to include all minor uterine cavity abnormalities

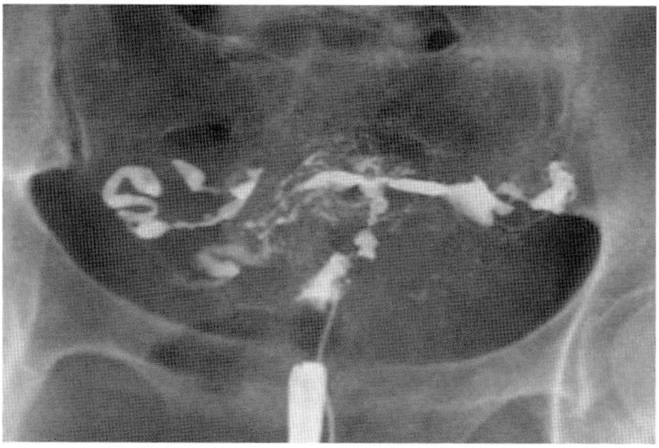

Fig. 5.6 HSG showed the characteristic features of T-shaped, narrow, and irregular uterine cavity

5.2.2 Indications

1. Unlike other uterine anomalies, a T-shaped uterus due to DES exposure during pregnancy can produce a full-term pregnancy. Therefore, not all patients diagnosed with T-shaped uterus require surgery, but then patients may have a history of adverse pregnancy outcome such as spontaneous miscarriage, premature birth, etc., and after excluding other causes of miscarriage, hysteroscopic corrective surgery is the appropriate treatment.
2. Intrauterine adhesions can also cause T-shaped uterus. If the narrow uterine cavity and endometrial damage lead to scanty menstruation, miscarriage, and other adverse pregnancy outcomes, hysteroscopic surgery may be required.
3. Patients with DES exposure in utero might have cervical incompetence due to abnormal uterine and cervical anomalies. During pregnancy, bed rest and preventive or emergency cervical cerclage might be needed to avoid midtrimester miscarriage and premature birth. Therefore, it had been suggested that in DES-exposed pregnant women, prophylactic cervical cerclage should be performed during pregnancy. However, prophylactic cervical cerclage during pregnancy is still controversial, and further RCT studies will be needed [18, 26].

5.2.3 Timing of Surgery

Hysteroscopic surgery should be offered to patients with T-shaped uterine cavity and a history of infertility or adverse pregnancy outcomes. It can also be used to treat patients who failed IVF-ET treatment. Surgery can be performed soon after menstruation to avoid a thickened endometrium which might impact on the hysteroscopic surgery.

5.2.4 Contraindications

1. It is important to exclude other factors leading to infertility, recurrent miscarriage, and premature labor. Then hysteroscopic surgery can be chosen to treat this uterine factor that is responsible for the adverse pregnancy outcomes. Otherwise, treatments should be directed to treat other relevant factors.
2. Patients with adhesion-induced T-shaped uterus, particularly those aged over 40 years of age, require a comprehensive assessment of their reproductive potential. Only after effective communication with patients should surgery be performed; otherwise, in patients without fertility issue or with no significant menstrual changes, there is no need for any surgery. Combined estrogen and progesterone therapy would be given if it is necessary.
3. Patients with T-shaped uterine cavity due to exposure to DES in utero do not require surgery if they have no history of adverse pregnancy outcome.

5.2.5 Preoperative Preparation

1. According to HSG or 3D ultrasound findings, the measurements of the distance between tubal openings, the depth of uterine cavity, and the bilateral and fundal myometrium thickness would give an assessment of the amount and depth of uterine wall excision during surgery.
2. Oral contraceptives can be used to control the endometrial thickness 1 month before the surgery.
3. Routine preoperative preparations are as other gynecological surgery. Twelve to twenty-four hours before the surgery, softening of the cervix by insertion of a laminaria tent might be useful as cervical preoperative treatment in some patients.

5.2.6 Anesthesia

Intravenous anesthesia or general anesthesia can be chosen. Patients should have vital signs and electrolytes monitoring so as to avoid the fluid overload "TURP" syndrome.

5.2.7 T-Shaped Uterine Cavity Surgery

Key surgical techniques for T-shaped uterine cavity hysteroscopic surgery [19, 27–29]:

1. Intraoperative ultrasound monitoring to increase the safety of the surgery.
2. Routine antiseptic preparation for the vulva and vagina should be taken. The cervix was dilated with dilators to the size of the operative hysteroscope.
3. Careful hysteroscopic examination to observe the positions of tubal openings, to correlate with the preoperative HSG and 3D ultrasound findings, and to assess the depth of uterine wall excision.
4. The resectoscope electrode needle should be positioned vertically to the lateral uterine wall below the fallopian tube opening. The uterine wall is incised from the fundus to the uterine isthmus; according to the preoperative and intraoperative assessment of the depth of uterine wall thickness, the first electrode which cut along the side wall of the uterus would create a groove from the fundus to the uterine isthmus; this will be performed again one to two times. It is important to control the depth of cutting, with deep cut initially, to shallow cut at the end. The cut depth should be controlled within 5–7 mm, to avoid surgical complications like uterine perforation or very thin myometrium. In the same way, the contralateral lateral wall of the uterus is cut; to assess the completeness of the procedure, the hysteroscope can be moved to the middle of the uterine cavity, in order to obtain a symmetrical inverted triangle view of the uterine cavity with bilateral easily observable tubal openings.
5. To prevent secondary intrauterine adhesions after surgery, an intrauterine balloon or IUCD can be inserted, and combined estrogen and progesterone cyclical treatment should be given to promote endometrial growth.
6. It must be emphasized that after two menstrual cycles, a repeat hysteroscopic examination is necessary to assess the effectiveness of the surgery and to assess whether there are recurrent adhesions, and if necessary, hysteroscopic adhesiolysis can be performed.

5.3 Bicornuate Uterus

Limin Feng

Congenital uterine anomalies have an overall incidence rate of 0.1–10 %; in pregnant women, it is 4.3 %; in infertile women, 3.5 %; and in women with recurrent miscarriage, 13 %. Therefore, the incidence of uterine anomalies is closely related to pregnancy outcome. The uterus is the place where the fertilized egg embeds and the fetus grows and develops. Therefore, abnormal uterine morphology and function is one of the primary reasons for infertility, miscarriage, premature delivery, intrauterine growth retardation, and obstructed labor.

Bicornuate uterus (also known as uterus bicornis) is a common symmetrical uterine anomaly caused by incomplete development of the paramesonephric duct. Its incidence is approximately 13.6 % of all uterine anomalies. During embryonic development, the two paramesonephric ducts, also known as Müllerian ducts, merge incompletely in the middle part and are not completely absorbed, therefore forming a cervix and two uterine cavities. The upper portion and the bottom portion of the uterine cavity appear like a fork. The tip of the unabsorbed partition is blunt and round. According to the Buttram classification, a bicornuate uterus is called a complete bicornuate uterus if it starts to divide the uterine cavity from the internal os of the cervix. On the other hand, it is an incomplete bicornuate uterus if it divides the cavity from anywhere above the internal os of the cervix. The two uterine horns can be at different distances from the internal cervical os. Their degrees of separation can also be different. There can be connections at different positions between the two uterine horns. The bicornuate uterus typically has more menstrual blood and different degrees of dysmenorrhea.

5.3.1 Clinical Manifestations

Some patients with minor degree of bicornuate uterus may not have any symptoms. Their menstruation, pregnancy, and childbirth may not show any obvious abnormalities. The bicornuate uterus in these patients is often incidentally found and diagnosed during examination. At menarche, some patients with bicornuate uterus may present with excessive menstruation and dysmenorrhea; women of childbearing age may present with infertility, recurrent miscarriages, and ectopic pregnancy; and fetal malposition during pregnancy especially breech presentation is most common. Due to poorly developed myometrium of the uterine horn, cervical dilatation may be slow, possibly leading to dystocia, uterine rupture, placenta retention, etc.

5.3.2 Diagnosis

1. For patients with a medical history of infertility, miscarriage, premature delivery, intrauterine growth retardation, or obstructed labor, there may be a possibility of uterine anomalies. Hence, further gynecological examinations and investigations are required.
2. Gynecological examination during nonpregnancy time may reveal two palpable horns of the bicornuate uterus. In early pregnancy, one horn may be enlarged by the pregnancy and the other horn shows hypertrophy.
3. Ultrasound examination: A 2D ultrasound examination can reveal a downward depression in the fundus of the uterus like the shape of a saddle. Three-dimensional ultrasound scan has overcome the limitations of two-dimensional ultrasound with regard to coronal images of the uterus and provides a more holistic, direct visualization of the morphology of the uterine fundus and endometrial cavity, resulting in a more objective and reliable diagnosis. Four-dimensional ultrasound as the latest ultrasound technology not only obtains accurate three-dimensional ultrasound images but also shows the status of uterine activity, to give a comprehensive and dynamic understanding of the uterus. The best time to perform ultrasound examination is at premenstrual period when the endometrium visualization is good and the uterine shape is easy to observe.
4. Hysterosalpingography: This method can show the location, size, shape of the uterine cavity and fallopian tube and can better show the majority of uterine anomalies. It is therefore the main diagnostic method for uterine malformations.
5. Imaging examination: CT scan has short imaging time, has high spatial resolution, and produces clear anatomical images. It is consistently reliable and it allows easy comparison between images of the complete cervix and uterine body. However, it has low resolution on soft tissues; hence, the endometrium and myometrium are indistinguishable. Magnetic resonance imaging (MRI), on the other hand, can provide high-resolution images on the uterine body, the fundus of the uterus, and the internal structure. It has no ionizing radiation. It can diagnose most types of uterine anomalies and can even allow coexisting urinary tract abnormalities to be identified. However, it is a more expensive imaging method.
6. Endoscopic examination: Laparoscopy can provide direct observations on uterine morphology, and hysteroscopy can enable abnormalities in the uterine cavity to be detected. The combined use of both can assess the condition of the uterine cavity and uterine appearance. It is the gold standard for assessment of uterine anomaly and is the method of choice for subsequent surgical treatment.

5.3.3 Indication

Patients with fertility demand, infertility, poor obstetrics history, and suspected bicornuate uterus

5.3.4 Timing of Surgery

The operation should be performed 3–7 days after cessation of menstruation.

5.3.5 Contraindications

1. Patients with genital tract infections
2. Patients at the time of menstrual period
3. Patients who are medically not fit for surgery, for example, those with cardiac and pulmonary insufficiency, abnormal liver and kidney functions, and coagulation disorders
4. Patients who cannot tolerate general anesthesia

5.3.6 Preoperative Preparation

1. It is important to take a detailed medical history to exclude patients with contraindications for surgery.
2. In addition to the patient's medical history, proper physical body examination and appropriate laboratory investigations should be carried out to assess the risks. This surgery may involve both the uterine cavity and vagina which should be adequately cleansed and without infection. Any special or acute infection should be treated before the surgery. The various emergency situations and complications arising from the surgery should also be fully evaluated and contingency plans made.
3. Patient's preparation:

   (a) Mental preparation: The patient is informed of the purpose and significance of the surgery. A patient should resolve any concern of surgery through preoperative counseling and discussions. She should sign the informed consent for the surgery.
   (b) Preoperative preparations include routine preoperative laboratory test and bacterial culture for vaginal discharge. Abdominal skin preparation is for general abdominal surgery, with the umbilicus cleansed to prevent infection. Bowel preparation includes semisolid diet 1 day before surgery, no food nor water starting from 12 o'clock the night before surgery, and a routine enema in the morning. Appropriate sedative is given to ensure good quality of sleep and the bladder emptied before surgery.

5.3.7 Anesthesia

According to the degree of difficulty of the operation, appropriate anesthesia such as local anesthesia, spinal anesthesia, epidural anesthesia, or general anesthesia is to be chosen. General anesthesia with intubation is commonly used for this surgery.

5.3.8 Surgical Procedures and Techniques

1. The laparoscopic examination:

   After placement of the laparoscope, any pathology or lesions in the abdominal and pelvic organs are to be examined. As bicornuate uterus and other types of genital anomalies are often associated with urinary tract abnormalities, a comprehensive exploration is required to see if there are other abnormal or missing organs.

   Examination of all the pelvic organs will be performed with the help of a uterine manipulator. Careful inspections are necessary to assess the uterus, fallopian tubes, the shape and size of the ovaries and for the presence of any pelvic adhesions, with or without pelvic endometriosis, and finally for any dilated pelvic varicose veins. If the examination reveals abnormal lesions, the location, size, nature, and their relationship with the surrounding organs should be noted. The surgical indications and appropriate surgical methods should be appropriately determined.
2. The hysteroscopic examination: Under a direct laparoscopic monitoring, a hysteroscopy examination is performed to inspect the uterine cavity and confirm the diagnosis of a bicornuate uterus.
3. Combined laparoscopic and hysteroscopic surgery:

   (a) Hysteroscopic surgery: Under laparoscopic monitoring of the uterus, the uterine partition of the uterus is cut and divided with a hysteroscopic needle electrode. The muscular uterine wall in the middle of the fundal uterus is cut separated up to the serosal layer. An artificial perforation at the uterine fundus is then made (Fig. 5.7). The fundal cavity of the uterus and the abdominal cavity are now fully communicated (Fig. 5.8). The next step will involve returning back to the laparoscopic surgery. In recent years, a bipolar resectoscope that uses saline perfusion has become available and is used commonly. Its use will avoid hyponatremia and increase the safety of hysteroscopic surgery.

   (b) Laparoscopic surgery: Under a laparoscope, the fundal part of the uterus is opened horizontally by a unipolar scissor, resulting in a transverse uterine incision up to 1–1. 5 cm from the two horns (Fig. 5.9). The cut uterine wound is now vertically and interruptedly sutured using Vicryl/0 stitch to the whole layer of the uterine wall over the uterine fundus (Fig. 5.10a) and close the uterine cavity (Fig. 5.10b), hence completing the reconstruction and fusion of the uterine fundus. (Fig. 5.11). An Interceed anti-adhesive film is now placed on the fundal wound surface which will help to prevent adhesion formation with other abdominal organs.

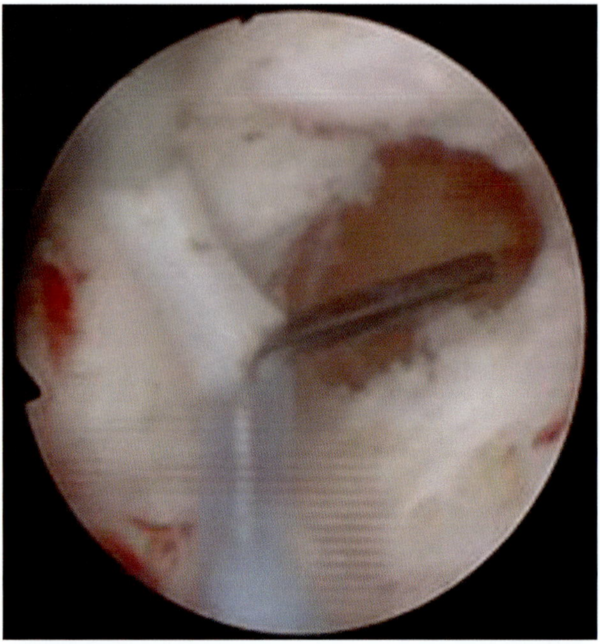

Fig. 5.7 An artificial perforation at the uterine fundus

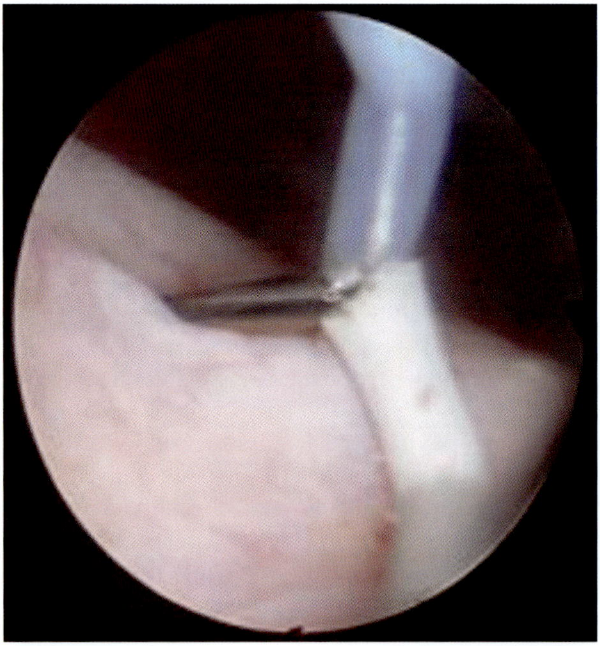

Fig. 5.8 Communicated uterus fundus and the abdominal cavity

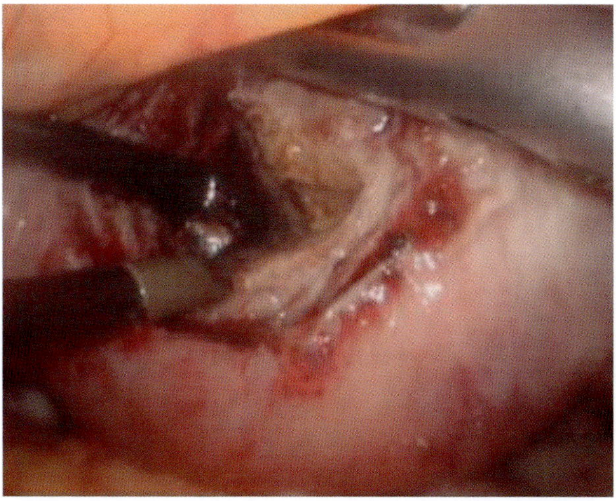

Fig. 5.9 The fundal part of the uterus is opened horizontally resulting in a transverse uterine incision up to 1–1.5 cm from the two horns

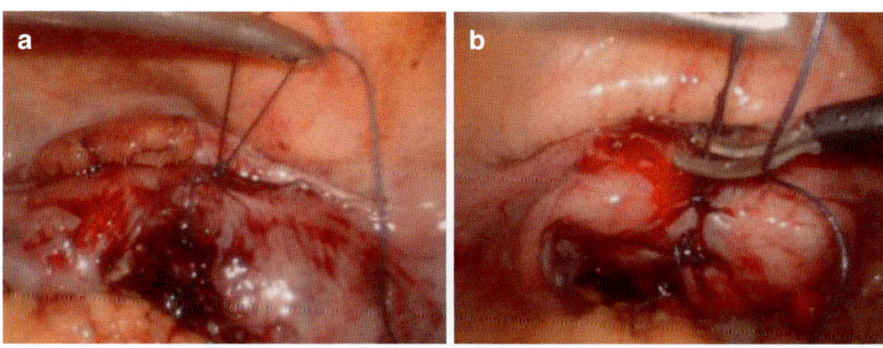

Fig. 5.10 The cut uterine wound is now vertically and interruptedly sutured using Vicryl /0 stitch to the whole layer of uterine wall over the uterine fundus (**a**) and close the uterine cavity (**b**)

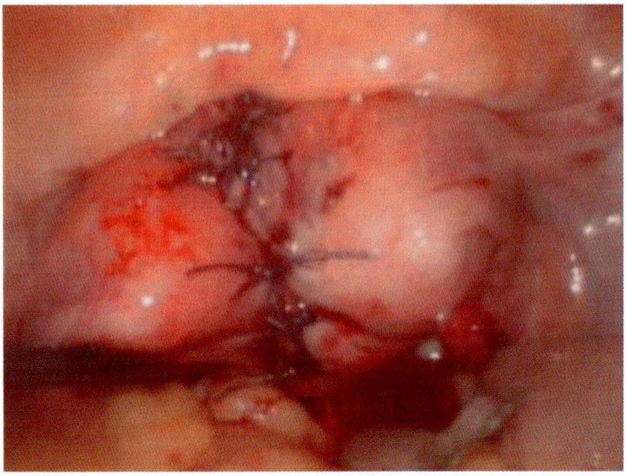

Fig. 5.11 The reconstruction and fusion of the uterine fundus

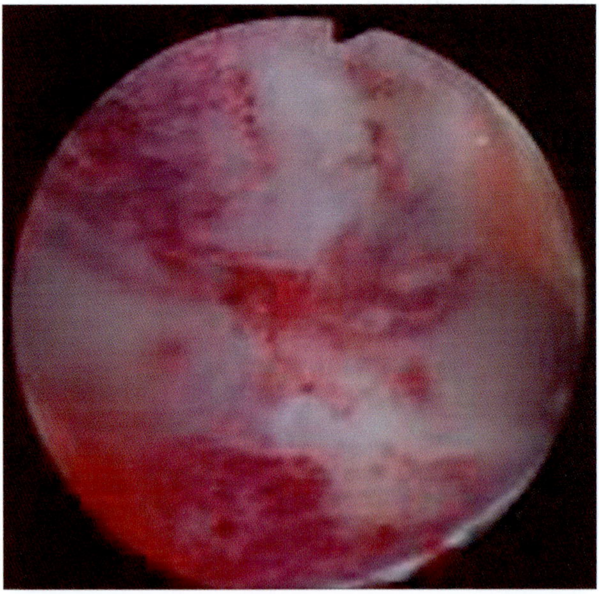

Fig. 5.12 The show with hysteroscopy 2 months after surgery

5.3.9 Key Points of Surgical Techniques

1. Key points of hysteroscopic surgical techniques
   (a) Hysteroscopic resection of the uterine partition: To remove the uterine partition with an electric needle electrode, the electric needle electrode is moved forward, i.e., a reverse cut to the direction of endometrium, unlike the resection of endometrium, endometrial polyps, or submucosal fibroids when the cutting is moved backward. Care must be taken not to harm the surrounding normal endometrium by electrical damage. The same should apply to avoid unintended uterine perforation resulting in injury to abdominal organs.
   (b) Complication prevention in hysteroscopic surgery: Complications of hysteroscopic surgery are uncommon, but if it happens, these may have some serious sequelae – uterine perforation, hyponatremia, bleeding, infection, and air embolism. Uterine perforation is the most common complication. If the activated electrical electrode passes through the uterine wall, it can harm neighboring organs. If the distending fluid using dextrose or glycine is overloaded, it can lead to hyponatremia. If injuries occur in the digestive tract, urinary tract, and large blood vessels, they can lead to fatal complications such as peritonitis, fistula, serious hemorrhage, and air embolism. Although the purpose of the hysteroscopic resection of the bicornuate uterus is to create an artificial perforation, care must be taken during surgery to avoid injury to the nearby organs and large blood vessels after the uterine perforation.
2. Postoperative management

   For the prevention of intrauterine adhesions after surgery, an intrauterine device (IUD) can be inserted into the uterine cavity together with oral estrogen and progesterone used for 2 months. After that, a second-look hysteroscopy examination should be performed (Fig. 5.12) to remove the IUD and assess the intrauterine condition. It is preferable that contraception be practiced and pregnancy avoided for at least 1 year.

5.3.10 Pregnancy After Surgery

Pregnancy in the bicornuate uterus is a high-risk pregnancy. It has a high rate of antenatal complications, labor dystocia, and operative delivery. This can lead to serious harm to the mother and the baby.

Some scholars believe that although the capacity of a malformed uterus to keep a pregnancy to full term is reduced, only when both the endometrium and myometrium have severe abnormal anomalies will this lead to infertility. Pedro Acien reported that the incidence of uterine anomalies is 0.1–2 %, but only 4 % of these people with uterine anomalies are infertile. This suggests that uterine anomalies would not significantly lead to infertility.

An abnormal uterus with pregnancy can easily lead to miscarriage or premature labor. Also, the incidences of fetal malposition and cesarean section significantly increase, and the average birth weight of newborns is reduced. These factors significantly increase the adverse pregnancy outcomes. Grimbizis reported the pregnancy outcome of 627 pregnancies in 260 patients with bicornuate uterus. The average abortion rate was 36 %, the average preterm delivery 23 %, full-term delivery 40.6 %, and average live birth 55.2 %. A retrospective study by China Union Medical College Hospital also showed that the bicornuate uterus can cause a variety of perinatal disorders such as recurrent miscarriage, premature labor, fetal malposition, fetal growth restriction, premature rupture of membrane, placenta previa, placental abruption, placenta accreta, fetal distress, secondary uterine atony, and postpartum hemorrhage.

Therefore, for patients with fertility demand and previous poor obstetric outcomes, a corrective surgery for bicornuate uterus during the nonpregnancy period should be performed. This may help to reduce the adverse pregnancy outcomes.

For patients with bicornuate uterus, there is still a lack of large and multicentre observational studies both at home and abroad with regard to their postoperative pregnancy outcome reported that abdominal hysteroplasty could significantly improve the pregnancy outcomes for those patients with recurrent spontaneous miscarriage or preterm delivery. After surgery, the full-term pregnancy rate could reach 90 %.

Reported that in 22 patients who had undergone laparoscopic uteroplasty for bicornuate uterus, 88 % had successful pregnancy and normal delivery also confirmed that, after laparoscopic uteroplasty, pregnancy to full term could reach 80–85 %.

Finally, there is an issue of concern which is the risk of scar rupture during pregnancy and at childbirth. According to in all their cases of cesarean section, there was no evidence of scar rupture, and some patients even showed no obvious scar in the uterus. Due to the rarity of bicornuate horn pregnancy, there are no reported guidelines for childbirth and delivery. Durok A et al. 2013 had recommended that planned elective cesarean section for this group of patients can reduce obstetric complications.

5.4 Uterine Septum

Xue Xiang

Uterine septum is the most common congenital uterine anomaly, being 80–90 % of all uterine anomalies. When the paramesonephric (Müllerian) ducts after fusion have reabsorption disorders, this will result in the formation of uterine septum due to incomplete cavitation preventing the formation of a single uterine cavity. Uterine septum is divided into two types: (a) complete septate uterus (Fig. 5.13), with septum reaching the internal os or sometimes ending outside the cervix, looking like a double cervix, and (b) incomplete uterine septum (Fig. 5.14), with septum ending in the cavity above the internal os of the cervix. Many uterine septa are incomplete uterine septum, and another 20–25 % of uterine septum are also associated with a vaginal longitudinal and oblique septum (Fig. 5.15).

The clinical manifestation of uterine septum is due to a ridge of connective tissue protruding into the uterine cavity with deep double uterine horns; as a result, the uterine cavity is relatively small. It is closely related to high rate of pregnancy failure, recurrent miscarriage, premature delivery, fetal malposition, intrauterine growth retardation, and other obstetric complications and infertility. But not all uterine septa affect fertility and obstetric outcomes; they depend on the length of the septum and the blunt or sharp edge of the septum (Fig. 5.16).

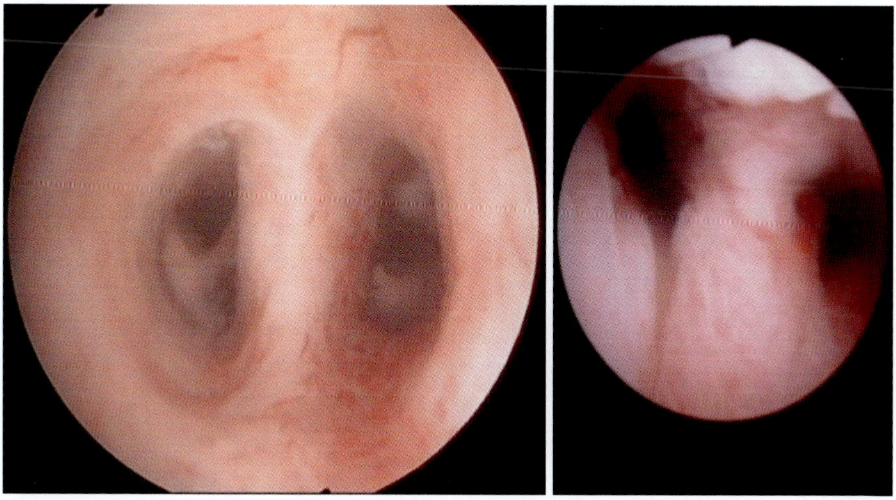

Fig. 5.13 Complete uterine septum with the septum reaching the internal cervical os

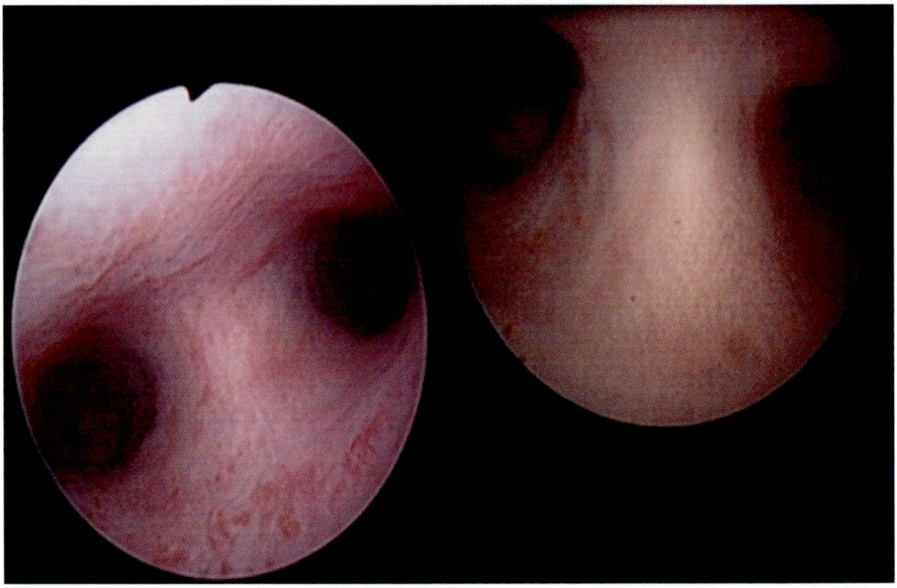

Fig. 5.14 Incomplete uterine septum, with fundal septum and bilateral deep uterine horn

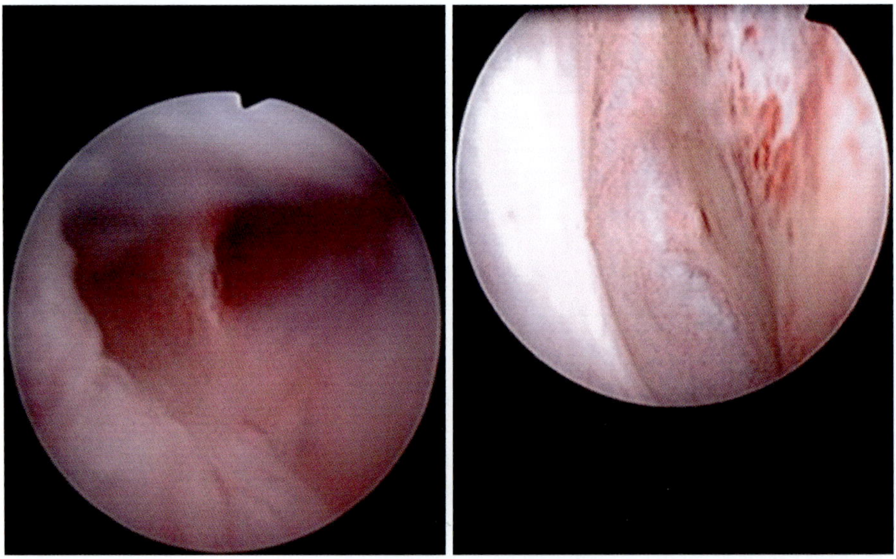

Fig. 5.15 Longitudinal vaginal septum or oblique vaginal septum associated with complete uterine septum

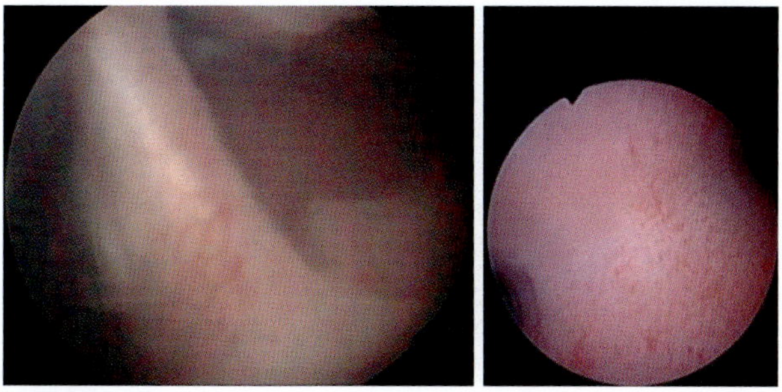

Fig. 5.16 Uterine septum with sharp edge and uterine septum with blunt thick edge

5.4.1 Diagnosis

The diagnostic methods for septate uterus include imaging studies and direct visual examination. In the past, patients with septate uterus presented with occult symptoms with its diagnosis easily missed. Often it was noticed and diagnosed after some pregnancy complications or reproductive disorders. With recent developments in hysterosalpingography (HSG), ultrasonography, hysteroscopy, laparoscopy, and magnetic resonance imaging (MRI) investigations, septate uterus has been increasingly diagnosed.

These investigations have their own diagnostic advantages as follows: HSG can display uterine cavities in both horns on each side of the uterine septum, the length of the septum, and the patency of the fallopian tubes. However, the external shape of the uterus remains unclear. Ultrasound can measure the length of the septum for quantitative research, to define the morphology of the uterus. But it is sometimes difficult to distinguish between complete and incomplete uterine septum. It is however a reliable method to diagnose uterine abnormality. In our study, hysteroscopy could make a diagnostic accuracy in 97.3 % of cases, which is significantly higher than HSG and ultrasonography (ref). But hysteroscopy cannot observe the outer morphology of the uterus. If ultrasound or laparoscopy can combine with hysteroscopy, this can further improve the accuracy of diagnosis.

5.4.2 Indication

Many septate uteri do not affect fertility, and hence they do not require surgery. However, when the septum does impact on fertility or obstetric outcome, surgical treatment is the only method to correct the septum and should be implemented.

5.4.3 Timing of Surgery

Surgery should be performed 3–7 days after the menstruation to avoid any thickened endometrium.

5.4.4 Contraindications

1. Patients with genital tract infections
2. Patients during a menstrual period
3. Patients with medical diseases who are not suitable for surgery, e.g., those with heart or lung failure, liver or kidney disorders, as well as bleeding tendency

5.4.5 Preoperative Preparation

1. Full preoperative examinations and investigations are performed to exclude surgical contraindications.
2. Preoperative counseling and education, to make patients' coping better with the surgery and if any, with the complications. On the night before surgery, soft diet is allowed. No food or drink for 6 h is recommended before the surgery. Cleansing enema is given to prepare the bowel, and the umbilicus is cleaned for the laparoscopic surgery.
3. Vaginal preparation: Vaginal scrub with 0.5 % povidone-iodine solution, once a day, should be recommended for 3 days before surgery.
4. Cervical preparation: Adequate preoperative cervical preparation is essential. The commonly used method is that in the night before surgery, a cervical dilation rod such as a laminaria tent is inserted to soften the cervix. This helps to reduce the risk of cervical laceration during surgery, thus reducing the operative difficulty.

5.4.6 Anesthesia

General anesthesia is used if combined laparoscopy and hysteroscopy procedure of septum resection is to be performed. If hysteroscopic resection of septum alone is to be performed under ultrasound monitoring, epidural or general anesthesia can be used.

5.4.7 Surgical Procedures

1. Resection of an incomplete uterine septum
   (a) Hysteroscopic examination: The cervix is dilated up to Hegar dilator No. 9.5. A hysteroscope is inserted to give a clear understanding of the shape of the uterine cavity and locate the bilateral fallopian tube openings. An incomplete septum has the following hysteroscopic feature: abnormal uterine morphology with a septum visible from the uterine fundus to a position above the internal cervical os, dividing the uterine cavity into left and right parts. In each uterine part, there is only one fallopian tube opening.
   (b) Use a needle electrode to cut the lower end of the uterine septum, moving from bottom-up, alternating from the left to the right and back, to create a cavity by opening the septum up to the uterine fundus.

(c) Repeat hysteroscopic examination to inspect the uterine cavity. If the uterine cavity appears normal, both openings of the fallopian tubes can be seen from the same cavity. Also, there should be no active bleeding from the cavity.
(d) The procedure is completed after an IUCD is inserted into the new uterine cavity. The IUCD is removed at the time of examination after 3 months.

2. Resection of a complete uterine septum

(a) If there is an associated vaginal septum, it should be first removed.
(b) After the cervix is adequately exposed, uterine sound is used to explore both uterine cavities on both sides of the septum. The cavities are dilated separately and any communicating opening between the cavities is to be noted. For septum with a communicating channel, the cutting is to start from the level of the internal cervical os and move upward for the septum resection. For septum without a communicating channel, i.e., the two uterine cavities are not connected, a uterine dilator or a Foley balloon is placed in the contralateral uterine cavity serving as an indicator. The septum is cut open to enlarge the two uterine cavities into one and complete the septum resection. The cervical septum should be retained within the cervix.

Also if available, resection of uterine septum can be performed under laparoscopic or ultrasound monitoring in order to reduce the operative risk of perforation and increase the success rate of the operation.

Postoperatively an IUCD is inserted, together with combined estrogen and progesterone treatment which is administered for 3 months. Hysteroscopic appearance of the uterine cavity after 3 weeks and three months to evaluate the uterine recovery after surgery is shown in Figs. 5.17 and 5.18. The IUCD is removed at the time of examination after 3 months.

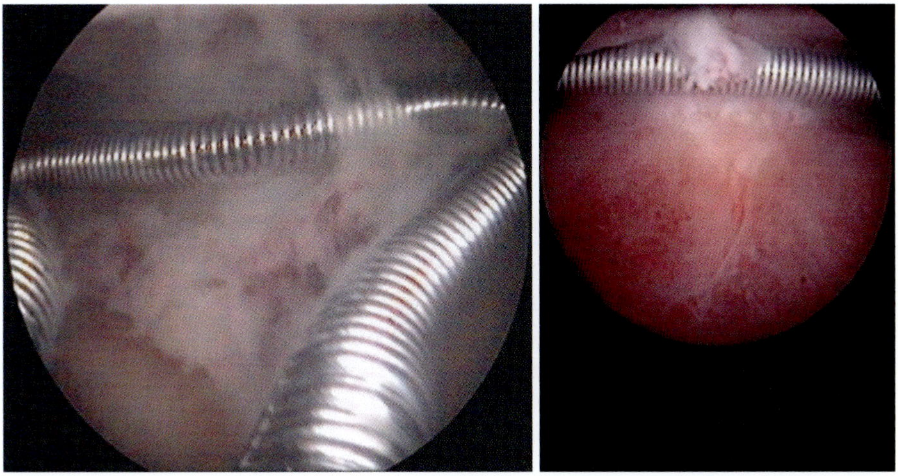

Fig. 5.17 Hysteroscopic appearance of the uterine cavity 3 weeks after septum resection

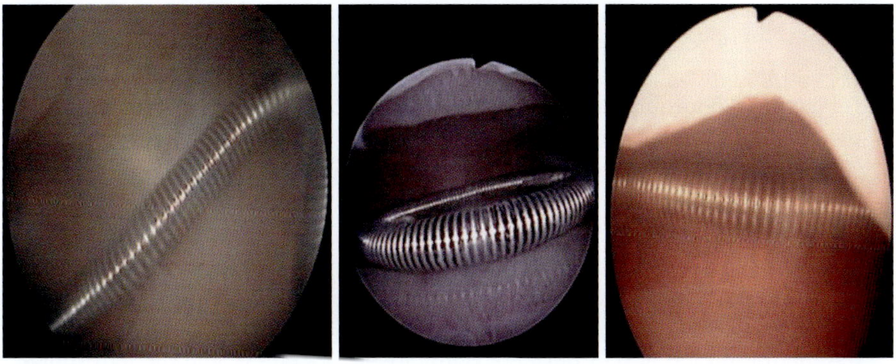

Fig. 5.18 Hysteroscopic appearance of the endometrial cavity 3 months after septum resection

5.4.8 Surgical Techniques

Hysteroscopic resection of the uterine septum is a reconstructive surgery. The surgery is intended to remove the septum in order to reduce its adverse impact on pregnancy and childbirth. It is also important to avoid any unnecessary damage to the uterine endometrium and any uterine perforation.

The key points of the surgical techniques are summarized as follows:

1. Either needle or curve electrodes can be chosen. The operative electrode is kept close to the center of the septum. Cutting toward the anterior or posterior walls of the uterus should be avoided in order to minimize injury to the uterine myometrium.
2. Timely halt cutting of the septum is recommended to avoid damaging the underlying myometrium. In controlling the depth of cutting, the following surgical indicators may be useful: when the cutting of the septum is near the uterine fundus, the hysteroscope can be moved in the new uterine cavity from one side to the other side; the hysteroscope can also show both bilateral fallopian tube openings; under the laparoscopic monitoring, the light transmission test from the uterine fundus should be uniform. Also if intraoperative ultrasonic monitoring is being used, when the distance between the cutting end and the serosal layer of the uterine fundus is approximately 1 cm, the septum cutting should be stopped. If bleeding noticeably increases at the cut surface, the cutting may have reached the myometrium and should be stopped.
3. Avoid injury to the cervix: As patients with septate uterus may have fertility demands, in order to avoid cervical insufficiency after surgery (which may lead to abortion and premature delivery), the transcervical resection surgery for a complete septum should cut and remove the septum tissue starting at the internal os of the cervix and moving upward away from the cervix.
4. Intraoperative monitoring: Combined laparoscopy and ultrasound monitoring of the septum resection will raise the safety of the operation, and the most important of all, it is to prevent uterine perforation.

5.4.9 Pregnancy After Septum Resection

Whether a septate uterus would affect a pregnancy depends on where the embryo embeds. Clinically, although not every septate uterus will cause pregnancy failure or infertility, nevertheless recurrent miscarriages and infertility are high in those with septate uterus, and thus significant improvements in achieving a good pregnancy outcome can be gained by septum resection. This indicates that surgical correction for a symptomatic septate uterus is an essential treatment. Compared with traditional open surgery, hysteroscopic septum resection not only removes the septum but also restores the normal morphology of the uterine cavity. At the same time, it leaves no surgical scar in the uterus and the abdomen. After operation, recurrence is low and recovery is fast. After hysteroscopic resection of the septum, the healing of the uterine wound will take about 2–3 months to complete. About 3 months after surgery, patient can be allowed to get pregnant. The peak time of pregnancy is from six months to a year after surgery. To summarize, hysteroscopic transcervical resection of uterine septum (TCRS) is safe and effective, and it can improve the pregnancy rate and outcome in these patients. It is therefore the preferred method of treatment for uterine septum. Xue Xiang et al. reported 118 cases of hysteroscopic resection of uterine septum from June 2006 to December 2010 for patients with infertility or recurrent miscarriages. For the infertility group, the pregnancy rate of patients after surgery increased to 51.9 %; full-term pregnancy was 29.6 %. For the recurrent abortion group, the spontaneous abortion rate decreased from 92.3 to 34.5 %; live birth increased from 66.7 to 95.6 %. There were significant differences compared to these patients before their surgeries. Since hysteroscopic uterine septum resection surgery does not destroy the integrity of the uterine wall and leaves no scar on the myometrium, the uterus is able to tolerate the uterine distension at pregnancy and to accommodate the contraction force at childbirth. The incidence of uterine rupture at pregnancy is low. Therefore, cesarean section is no longer essential as a conventional mode of delivery. The pregnancy outcome in patients after hysteroscopic septum resection has no significant difference compared with the control group with normal uterus. The complications of pregnancy, fetal development, perinatal mortality, and other indicators also show no difference between the two groups.

However, if the operation is not operated skillfully, resulting in the damage to the myometrium at the fundus or causing a uterine perforation without prompt recognition, then the risk of uterine rupture is likely to increase. Therefore, any pregnant women after transcervical resection of septum should be closely monitored during pregnancy and in labor, to ensure the safety of the mother and the child.

References

Rudimentary Horn

1. Chan YY, et al. The prevalence of congenital uterine anomalies in unselected and high-risk populations: a systematic review. Hum Reprod Update. 2011;17(6):761–71.
2. Reichman D, Laufer MR, Robinson BK. Pregnancy outcomes in unicornuate uteri: a review. Fertil Steril. 2009;91(5):1886–94.
3. Khati NJ, Frazier AA, Brindle KA. The unicornuate uterus and its variants: clinical presentation, imaging findings, and associated complications. J Ultrasound Med. 2012;31(2):319–31.
4. Grimbizis GF, et al. The ESHRE/ESGE consensus on the classification of female genital tract congenital anomalies. Hum Reprod. 2013;28(8):2032–44.
5. Bermejo C, et al. Three-dimensional ultrasound in the diagnosis of Mullerian duct anomalies and concordance with magnetic resonance imaging. Ultrasound Obstet Gynecol. 2010;35(5):593–601.
6. Trad M, Palmer S. Mullerian duct anomalies and a case study of unicornuate uterus. Radiol Technol. 2013;84(6):571–6.
7. Grimbizis GF, Campo R. Clinical approach for the classification of congenital uterine malformations. Gynecol Surg. 2012;9(2):119–29.
8. Melissa Blyth AG, Penketh R. Torsion of a rudimentary horn pregnancy – an unusual case presentation. Gynecol Surg. 2013;10(1):91–2.
9. Mavrelos D, et al. Ultrasound diagnosis of ectopic pregnancy in the non-communicating horn of a unicornuate uterus (cornual pregnancy). Ultrasound Obstet Gynecol. 2007;30(5):765–70.
10. Siwatch S, et al. Rudimentary horn pregnancy: a 10-year experience and review of literature. Arch Gynecol Obstet. 2013;287(4):687–95.
11. Shahid A, et al. Laparoscopic management of a 16-week ruptured rudimentary horn pregnancy: a case and literature review. Arch Gynecol Obstet. 2010;282(2):121–5.
12. Medeiros LR, et al. Laparoscopic approach of a unicornuate uterus with noncommunicating rudimentary horns. ISRN Obstet Gynecol. 2011;2011:906138.
13. Fedele L, et al. Laparoscopic removal of the cavitated noncommunicating rudimentary uterine horn: surgical aspects in 10 cases. Fertil Steril. 2005;83(2):432–6.
14. Vallerie AM, Breech LL. Update in Mullerian anomalies: diagnosis, management, and outcomes. Curr Opin Obstet Gynecol. 2010;22(5):381–7.
15. Spitzer RF, Kives S, Allen LM. Case series of laparoscopically resected noncommunicating functional uterine horns. J Pediatr Adolesc Gynecol. 2009;22(1):e23–8.
16. Letterie GS. Management of congenital uterine abnormalities. Reprod Biomed Online. 2011;23(1):40–52.

T-shaped Uterus

17. Herbst AL, Ulfelder H, Poskanzer DC. Adenocarcinoma of the vagina. Association of maternal stilbestrol therapy with tumor appearance in young women. N Engl J Med. 1971;284(15):878–81.
18. Goldberg JM, Falcone T. Effect of diethylstilbestrol on reproductive function. Fertil Steril. 1999;72(1):1–7.
19. Fernandez H, et al. Surgical approach to and reproductive outcome after surgical correction of a T-shaped uterus. Hum Reprod. 2011;26(7):1730–4.
20. Buttram Jr VC, Gibbons WE. Mullerian anomalies: a proposed classification. (An analysis of 144 cases). Fertil Steril. 1979;32(1):40–6.

21. The American Fertility Society classifications of adnexal adhesions, distal tubal occlusion, tubal occlusion secondary to tubal ligation, tubal pregnancies, mullerian anomalies and intrauterine adhesions. Fertil Steril. 1988;49(6):944–55.
22. Grimbizis GF, et al. The ESHRE/ESGE consensus on the classification of female genital tract congenital anomalies. Hum Reprod. 2013;28(8):2032–44.
23. Kaufman RH, et al. Continued follow-up of pregnancy outcomes in diethylstilbestrol-exposed offspring. Obstet Gynecol. 2000;96(4):483–9.
24. Kipersztok S, et al. Comparison of magnetic resonance imaging and transvaginal ultrasonography with hysterosalpingography in the evaluation of women exposed to diethylstilbestrol. J Reprod Med. 1996;41(5):347–51.
25. Grimbizis GF, Campo R. Clinical approach for the classification of congenital uterine malformations. Gynecol Surg. 2012;9(2):119–29.
26. Levine RU, Berkowitz KM. Conservative management and pregnancy outcome in diethylstilbestrol-exposed women with and without gross genital tract abnormalities. Am J Obstet Gynecol. 1993;169(5):1125–9.
27. Giacomucci E, et al. Term delivery rate after hysteroscopic metroplasty in patients with recurrent spontaneous abortion and T-shaped, arcuate and septate uterus. Gynecol Obstet Invest. 2011;71(3):183–8.
28. Garbin O, et al. Hysteroscopic metroplasty in diethylstilboestrol-exposed and hypoplastic uterus: a report on 24 cases. Hum Reprod. 1998;13(10):2751–5.
29. Katz Z, et al. Beneficial effect of hysteroscopic metroplasty on the reproductive outcome in a 'T-shaped' uterus. Gynecol Obstet Invest. 1996;41(1):41–3.

Index

© Springer Science+Business Media Dordrecht 2015

L. Zhu et al. (eds.), *Atlas of Surgical Correction of Female Genital Malformation*,
DOI 10.1007/978-94-017-7246-4

Printed by Printforce, the Netherlands